DELiVERiNG HOPE

The Extraordinary Journey
of a Surrogate Mom

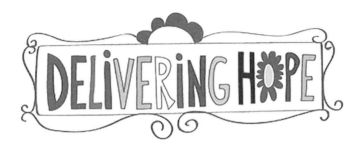

The Extraordinary Journey of a Surrogate Mom.

By Pamela MacPhee

Deliveringhopebook.com

Delivering Hope: The Extraordinary Journey of a Surrogate Mom
By Pamela A.B. MacPhee

Photo credits Robert G. MacPhee and Pamela A.B. MacPhee

Library of Congress Control Number: 2009924215

ISBN No. 978-0-615-28205-3

Published by HeartSet, Inc.
P.O. Box 232155
Encinitas, CA 92023

Printed in China

Design by Carolyn Gavin

FIRST EDITION

for kellie, duncan, lise

and my husband, robert,

who helped make the journey possible

Contents

THE WEEKEND GETAWAY
Calm Before the Storm...3

THE RIVER TRIP
Family Ties That Bind 15

THE DECISION
Choosing Surrogacy 33

THE CHINESE MAFIA
Preparing For Surrogacy 51

THE EMBRYO TRANSFER
Business or Pleasure?.. 67

THE FIRST TRIMESTER
Sharing the Pregnancy 89

THE SECOND TRIMESTER
This Baby Is Not Mine.. 115

THE THIRD TRIMESTER
The Baby is Coming 133

THE BIRTH
Hope Arrives 157

THE PARTY'S OVER
Restoration & Reflection... 191

EPILOGUE 206
PHOTOS 215

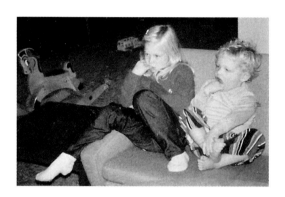

me & henry

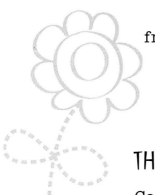

friday, may 11th, 2001

THE WEEKEND GETAWAY

Calm Before The Storm

SPRAWLED OUT ON MY BED in full pregnant splendor, I heard Mom and Dad pull into my driveway in coastal San Diego on a Friday afternoon. The kids dropped their books and commotion ensued as they ran around outside like racecars jostling for position to exchange warm hugs. I listened from my distant bedroom as Dad affectionately barked his familiar greetings,

"How are you, muscles?" he asked with a mischievous note in his voice. I could picture Mom with her eyebrows raised and her smile wide, as she made her hellos, searching for delight in the kids' eyes as confirmation of her arrival.

Smirking at the giggles and screams drifting in from outside, I heaved myself and my big pregnant belly up off the bed with a combination slide, push and grunt, my pathetic current version of the triathlon. I felt about as graceful as a rhinoceros rolling over. Just a few days shy of my due date, the fatigue of pregnancy had settled into my body as well as my mind. I stepped heavily through the halls and out the front door to welcome my parents, where the May afternoon air buzzed with the sounds and smells of spring and the excitement of family reconnecting.

"Great to see you, sweetheart, you look wonderful, are you feeling o.k.?" my mother inquired.

"Yep. I'm feeling really good, just big," I answered.

Mom and Dad appeared delighted to see me, relieved to reassure themselves in person that in the throes of this pregnancy I remained in reasonable physical and emotional health. As parents it is naturally their privilege and prerogative to worry about their children, and though at times I have been exasperated by their concern, secretly my siblings and I all feel lucky to be so cared for under their protection.

"Come on in everybody!" I invited.

My niece arrived in the company of my parents, and happily engaged in a tickling and chasing game with her younger cousins until they all eventually made their way inside, dragging suitcases, gifts, food and the odd assortment of bags and boxes that seems to follow my father wherever he travels. Mom and Dad had arrived weary from the eight-hour drive down from the Bay Area, but emerged reinvigorated from their exchange with their grandchildren. While they settled in and debated on where to unpack, I made my way back to my room to solve my own packing dilemma.

Desperately looking forward to a weekend getaway with my husband for some much needed time and space away from the frenetic pace of our daily lives, I hopelessly tried to decide what to pack for our adventure. Robert, a self-employed consultant, arrived home shortly from his office a few miles down the coast, and we finished throwing our things together as we made last minute preparations to hit the road.

"We're fine here, you guys should get going," my Dad encouraged, happily looking forward to some rare time alone with his grandchildren.

Mom surprised me with a beautiful leather purse before we stepped out the door, a generous gift which I happily carried with me for our weekend adventure. My mother delights in bestowing gifts upon her children and grandchildren, seldom bothering to wrap them or (to my dad's dismay) to even take off the price tags, and always eager to press them into our hands, tokens of her love and generosity of spirit.

After a barrage of hugs, kisses and earnest promises from our three little ones to be good, Robert and I exited the driveway, honking our horn goodbye and leaving the kids in the capable hands of my parents.

"Goodbye, Mommy! Goodbye, Daddy!" Kellie(8), Duncan(6), and Lise(3) shouted, waving happily as we drove away.

"Kellie, be a good girl, and help Boo and Papa John with your brother and sister!" I yelled out the window as they turned to walk inside.

Excited to share their most recent stories and treasures alone with their grandparents, they forgot about us before we even turned the corner. Easy going, well-adjusted kids, they exhibited no separation anxiety, no concern, confident that eventually we would be coming back.

I leaned back in the seat, exhaled exhaustedly and closed my eyes, enjoying the peacefulness of the breeze softly brushing my face and reveling in the time alone with Robert. Married eleven years, eight of them as parents of young children, we appreciated any time we could find alone for each other and the weekend ahead of us emerged like a precious gift. Inevitably, a subtle kick in the ribs from the lively bundle inside of me reminded me, however, that we were not truly alone; but that bundle could not talk back, at least not yet.

With a two-hour drive ahead of us up to Los Angeles, we took pleasure in the time to relax together in the relative quiet of the confines of our car and share our thoughts on the day. We could actually finish a conversation. Even Los Angeles traffic on a Friday afternoon does not feel like such a hellish zoo when you are busy cherishing a respite from the continuous effort required to be a parent.

Just a few short days away from completing nine months of my present pregnancy, I had chosen to pack the ubiquitous *What to Expect When You're Expecting* book right up front next to my feet, should I feel desperate to consult an authority when my anxieties about the delivery started to creep in.

I did not consider myself an accomplished pregnancy expert, even though this marked my fourth time around, because each of my previous deliveries had proven to be somewhat of a trial. Doctors delivered Kellie, my first, eight years earlier by way of a rather frightening emergency cesarean section after her head got stuck inside me and her heart rate dropped precipitously. Duncan arrived a year and a half later with a broken clavicle, poor little guy, after I narrowly avoided another emergency c-section. And Lise, weighing in at 9 pound 6 ounces, had entered the world with a brachial plexus nerve injury, a permanent limitation to the dexterity and range of motion of her left arm, which she suffered when the doctor wrongly applied excessive force to release her wedged shoulder.

Given my less than stellar history, I felt I deserved the right to panic, and the book acted as my crutch.

Since we would be out of San Diego County for the next 36 hours, Robert exhibited more than a little concern about his responsibility to get me back home in time to deliver the baby at our local hospital, should I go into labor.

"So what does it say in that book about delivering a baby in a car?" he inquired casually, although somewhat seriously, as we merged onto the 5 freeway heading North. He is a consummate planner who prefers to map out the near future in at least a general outline.

"Well, let's see," I began as I mockingly read to him from the *What to Expect* book about how to perform an emergency delivery in a motorized vehicle.

I teased him about being slightly paranoid, but I noticed we both listened intently to every word of that section, a few paragraphs which previously had prompted us to laugh at the idiots who would risk placing themselves in such a precarious situation. While not exhibiting any signs of going into labor, I had invited trouble by leaving town so soon before the baby's due date, and anxiety about the accompanying risk nagged at me uneasily.

The advice the book gives is practical, but not particularly realistic. The authors recommend you laid down towels to protect the surfaces of the car, but, I noted, that would necessitate precious time and a calm presence of mind during an emergency, not to mention the forethought required to pack a towel in the first place. Without any linens to speak of, our eyes rested on Robert's suit coat hanging in the back seat. I supposed it would be easier to dry clean his coat than scrub the leather seats clean of remnants of the birthing process, but I seriously doubted that he would ever feel comfortable sliding into the sleeves of that jacket again once it had been soaked through with blood and amniotic fluid.

The *What to Expect* book also emphasizes that it is the husband's job to soothe and reassure the panicking pregnant wife. I could just picture it:

"Oh, honey, I see the head starting to crown. I'll put on some James Taylor, recline the seats, open the moon roof, and look lovingly into your eyes!"

I've got to tell you neither of us retained any misconceptions about who would be calming who, given my husband's squeamishness about blood and pain. He passed out before our oldest daughter was even born, dragging the whole rolling epidural cart crashing to the floor with him, medical instruments skidding noisily in all directions. He'll tell you it's perfectly reasonable that watching the anesthesiologist's sterile needle poke repeatedly into my spinal column caused him to pass out, but I will only remind him that **I** was the one with that big old epidural needle jabbing into my back like a relentless wasp. And I was the one left alone, hunched over on the hospital bed rolling my eyes in pain (and frustration), while every nurse and doctor in the place tended to him splayed out on the floor.

"I'm here for you, honey!" he had called out weakly in a dazed voice from below me. Sure you are. Like a rock.

To be honest, though, Robert is strong for me when I am weak. His mere presence is calming and comforting to me, and I can not imagine delivering a baby without him at my side. He has a confident way with his sarcastic sense of humor and caring touch of burying my doubts as they creep into my consciousness, managing somehow to be a comfort even when he happens to be incapacitated and unconscious.

When we pulled up to the tollbooth for the 73 freeway through Orange County, Robert's sense of humor surfaced mischievously.

"Hey, can I ask you a question," Robert inquired of the toll taker.

"Sure," he answered.

"We were wondering if there had ever been a birth on the toll road?" Robert asked with a straight face, pointing to my alarmingly protruding belly.

"No. You guys would be the first," the guy assured us hesitantly with an anxious look at my midsection. Our ensuing sarcastic enthusiasm that we could be the first to deliver a baby on that stretch of asphalt, served to elicit a chuckle out of the lonely man in that tiny box.

To set the record straight about the rest of my *dream emergency car birth experience* (I think that's the definition of an oxymoron), I should let you know that the back seat did not recline, James Taylor remained silent on a dusty old LP in the attic, and the sun would have blinded me unrelentingly through the moon roof on that May afternoon. I, for one, given the opportunity to choose the birthing environment, would unquestionably prefer the sterile confines of a mundane hospital room over the cramped and littered backseat of our Audi. The 73 freeway is welcome to bestow upon some other unwitting pregnant couple the honor of *first roadside delivery*.

The only delivery I would have welcomed that afternoon comes served in neatly folded white cartons with a fortune cookie.

Our trip proved uneventful and we arrived at the funky Shangri La hotel in Santa Monica without any incident or unplanned deliveries. I indulged in the opportunity to be away from home with no immediate responsibilities, without the overwhelming demands of parenthood, instead with the freedom to lounge on the bed like a carefree teenager without the gravity of my belly weighing heavily on my tired legs. Robert, too, allowed himself to relax outside the magnetic draw of the work zip code.

After a brief rest, we showered and dressed for the rehearsal dinner of a close college friend, whose wedding the following evening had been our excuse to sneak away on this weekend together. We whisked off to Westwood (okay, I didn't really whisk, it was more like a slow stir) to the penthouse digs of the Regency Club.

Stepping off the elevator and into the foyer, turning head-on into the crowded room, or belly-on in my case, we failed miserably at any attempt to join the party inconspicuously. My belly pointed the way like a searchlight in a dark forest, forging a path to the outside balcony, where we tracked down the bride-to-be and her fiancé mingling dutifully.

"We are so excited for you both!" We congratulated them, shaking hands and hugging each other.

Stacey is one from my group of girlfriends with whom I had forged close ties when we studied abroad together at the Stanford campus in Florence, and the group of us have been sharing life's ups and downs on the backbone of our unspoken, unwavering support to each other ever since. Through broken hearts, career changes, marriage and childbirth, they have always been there; the kind of friends who will hold your hand when you are sick, let you know when you do something stupid, and tell someone else off if they have the audacity to hurt you. Stacey had waited patiently for her knight in shining armor, and we rejoiced in her happiness when he finally found her.

The overflowing joy of the newlywed-couple-to-be proved contagious, and we happily watched them be lured away from one well-wisher to the next like a well-orchestrated dance on that crowded deck. Robert and I were left standing alone to observe the other guests drift by, indulging in our relative anonymity. We felt like secret escapees to a foreign culture, the universe of Los Angeles, complete with its own set of planets revolving in unique orbital speeds and directions. Holding hands and sipping from our champagne glasses, we enjoyed the time alone in each other's company with a birds-eye view of the setting sun reflected in the windows of Westwood. Eventually, the bride's father flagged us down and engaged us in an entertaining repartee on his personal insights into Robert Redford and Hollywood moviemaking.

Stacey's mother, however, appeared to be rendered somewhat speechless when she laid her eyes on my swollen belly, mortified I would deliver right there on the penthouse buffet table sprawled out among the shrimp and fresh Italian mozzarella.

"My dear, are you o.k.? Are you sure you should be here?" she asked.

"I'm fine. The baby is quiet in my belly and I feel great," I reassured her, promising there would be no need for a 911 call before the final toasts were delivered on her daughter's big night.

A little later, as we prepared to devour the tantalizing treats we had loaded up on our dinner plates from the buffet, we maneuvered ourselves into our assigned seats at a table of the bride and groom's family and friends. To our delight we discovered our seats to be among a true cast of entertaining characters who conversed wittily from one engaging topic to another.

The friendly banter inevitably touched on my pregnancy, but I deflected the attention away, content to be a contributor to the conversation rather than a subject up for review. Our discussion that evening instead segued into an array of baby and sex topics; nothing was taboo by the end of the evening. In what has become a seemingly universal law, the presence of a pregnant woman gives people carte blanche to share the most intimate details of their own pregnancies and deliveries, and, emboldened by a few glasses of cabernet, our tipsy table-mates were even eager to share the private details of the fateful encounters that preceded the appearance of that telling red line on the pregnancy test stick.

The sexual banter continued all in good fun, though I imagine

Emily Post would have found our conversation shockingly lacking in appropriate social restraint and decorum, and we connected as a group while refraining from stepping over the line into the realm of sharing *too much information.*

While the buffet tables tempted us with luscious desserts after dinner, the bride's brothers regaled us with the requisite silly speeches and touching toasts before guests made their way up to thank the hosts and head home for the night. Stacey's mother appeared relieved to conclude the evening without any maternity emergencies. Robert and I left the party remarkably relaxed, having delighted in sharing such a special night with a dear friend and with each other, and thankful for a shift in attention away from the pregnancy and impending arrival of the baby. Though tired, I slipped into a warm contentment as I gazed out my passenger window into the mesmerizing evening lights of Sunset Boulevard.

Saturday morning arrived, lazy and unhurried, and we slept in for the first time in months, waking up leisurely to the remarkable absence of shouted whispers, blaring cartoons, and clanging cereal bowls. We love our children and can't imagine life without them, but though they are our pride and joy, a short break is never unappreciated. In fact, I think it makes us better parents. Allowing us to reconnect with each other and ourselves energizes us, making us better equipped to respond intelligently, reasonably, compassionately to the kids' needs and to appreciate each of them fully: Kellie's intellect and maturity, Duncan's caring side in the midst of his boisterous boyishness, and Lise's compassion and sensitivity.

Following a couple of long, hot showers, we checked out of the hotel and meandered along in search of a hearty breakfast to satisfy our growing appetites. Taking the time to absorb the Saturday newspaper over croissants, eggs, bacon and fresh orange juice at a local eatery, we wandered afterward in search of shops on a quest for a few small treasures, and found ourselves strolling through the local farmers market, where we purchased blood oranges from a heaping pile for the wedding couple.

After delivering the fresh fruit to the doorstep of the new home where Stacey and her fiancé would begin their adventure as husband and wife, we cruised in the car through twists and turns down into Beverly Hills, and later napped on the beach back in Santa Monica, listening to the background hush of the ocean waves breaking as they met the sandy shore. The anticipation of the approaching birth hovered just beneath the surface of our conversation, gathering momentum with every passing hour until the time when it would break the silence like those waves upon the sand.

The salty smell of the surf and the cool touch of the ocean spray acted as a tonic for my mind and body, as I lay there reflecting about the wonder of the life inside of me, imagining how my perspective would shift giving birth to this baby. The sun's approach to the horizon signaled the end of a treasured day of down time with Robert; a day that had served to restore our inner strength in preparation for the physical and emotional effort to bring a new child into the world.

Shifting gears from our relative anonymity and solitude, Robert and I hurried up to the front door of my cousin's home in Manhattan Beach to change for Stacey's wedding.

"Hey guys, come on in," my cousin, Henry, and his wife, Lauren, greeted us warmly, gazing distractedly at my round belly.

"How's that baby doing?" Henry inquired raptly.

I gently placed his hand and Lauren's on top of the bulge in my maternity shirt in an effort to connect them through the barriers of clothing, skin and amniotic fluid with the precious life cradled in my belly.

Their fingers lingered there hopefully, searching for evidence of the life inside of me whose pulsing blood carried their genes. This baby, their baby, encompassed the dreams they hoped to fulfill in becoming a family and they had patiently waited nine long months while I carried her inside me as a surrogate mother; waited for the day when their biological connection would become a tangible presence they could cradle and comfort outside the separation imposed by my uterus.

This baby inside me belonged to Lauren and to Henry, my mother's sister's son, my childhood companion. The baby was not mine.

"Sorry you guys, she's not moving right now. I think the sounds of the waves rocked her to sleep," I apologized.

Without feeling any detectable movement, Lauren and Henry reluctantly slid their hands off my belly, ushering Robert and me into the guest bedroom to transform ourselves from casual weekend beachgoers into elegant wedding party guests.

But first I could not resist sneaking a peek at the nursery Henry and Lauren had decorated in expectation of the arrival of their infant daughter. I carried my big old belly up the stairs and tread gently into the baby's room, which they had, to my delight, gussied up into a chamber fit for a princess. I curled my toes into the soft white carpet while I gazed around the adorable space, smiling contentedly at the waiting crib, the diapers lined up at the changing table, and the drawers full of tiny onesies, silky dressing gowns and cuddly receiving blankets.

The visible evidence of their loving preparation for the baby curled up inside my belly gently comforted me. I had offered to fulfill the role of a surrogate when doctors declared Lauren physically incapable of carrying a child, and following a year-long journey of surrogacy, highlighted by a successful frozen embryo transfer, Henry and Lauren could now look forward to the joy of becoming parents.

Imagining the baby inside me snuggled into their arms as they rocked her gently in the cozy space of that room, I cherished expectantly her tenderly awaited arrival into their family. Fading light stirred through the West window, softly filling the room heavy with hope and anticipation for a baby girl.

I would be relinquishing my role as caretaker and safe haven for Henry and Lauren's daughter, when I delivered her into this world for them in a matter of hours. As I stood there silently in the nursery, the baby resting peacefully inside me, I took pleasure in the accomplishment of navigating a long obstacle course toward reaching a common goal, savoring my delight in the moment and the magnitude of the gift I would be giving my cousin.

And I wondered what it would actually feel like to give birth to someone else's child, to hand over a baby I had nourished inside me for nine long months to another set of parents. What would I be left with?

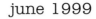

june 1999

THE RIVER TRIP

Family Ties That Bind

ROBERT AND I WERE INVITED two years earlier, along with my siblings and cousins, to join our parents for a week long adventure of family bonding amidst one of nature's most inspiring displays of raw beauty and grandeur, The Grand Canyon.

My mom and her sister are intimate friends despite their different personalities, and though my Aunt Pam is more of the independent thrill-seeking-do-it-yourselfer while my mother is more the supportive encouraging-people-person, they are both positive individuals with a great love for life, and for living it fully. Delighting in bringing our families together to encourage our mutual friendship and connection, with their husbands as willing partners they had planned a river rafting trip for all of us through the center of one of the natural Wonders of the World.

With the kids well taken care of at home by a competent babysitter, we arrived on a remote patch of dirt on the North side of the Canyon, hundreds of miles removed from the crowds incessantly snapping pictures along the railings of the South Rim. There, in the searing dry heat of June, after a night at the local motel, twelve family members among a group of twenty-seven travelers boarded sturdy rafts and floated away from the shore, submerged nets stocked full of Gatorade trailing behind us like a kite's tail, beginning our journey into the depths of the Grand Canyon.

"O.k. we're off!" our guides exalted. Within minutes we had spotted eagles nesting in trees lining the shore and marveled at the majesty of the canyon walls rising around us.

As I perused the eager faces in the raft surrounding me, it occurred to me that this would be our first extended family adventure since all us cousins had grown up together as rowdy young kids, clambering up the rocky trails on backpacking trips into the Desolation Wilderness long before Robert had married into this mess. Though each of us is unique in our own special way (read: strange, particular, peculiar), we are bonded together now by family ties and shared history into a loosely cohesive mass of relatively well-adjusted (though often juvenile) group of adults.

Of course, we had all gone through our *phases* in the interim. There is my older sister, Marlene, the self-proclaimed vegetarian in college, who now stomps around in the woods shooting elk, supplying the rest of the family with meat for the winter. My younger sister, Heidi, best remembered as a child for singing the "Enjoli" perfume commercial while standing on the dining room table, now sells expensive dining room tables to sit at as an interior designer and frequently refrains from joining in on "Happy Birthday". My brother, Chris, on the other hand, has steered a steady, consistent course since childhood, intelligently escaping his three crazy sisters and extended family in the Bay Area to live in Tahoe City, where he speeds down the moguls on the quiet ski slopes and bakes up a storm in the oven in his spare time.

My cousin, Wende, followed Marlene's footsteps in college, embracing vegetarianism and subsequently proceeding to fade away before our eyes, refusing to eat much of anything, but who now, like my brother, scrapes a mean spatula in the kitchen as a gourmet cook on the side.

And then there is Wende's brother, my cousin, Henry, four years my junior. Though my earliest memories of him are as a very young child running around the house screaming like a banshee, destroying everything in his wake, he is now a meticulous organizer who cannot stand a mess, whether it is on a child's face or his living room floor. But he retained his curiosity, his spirit of adventure that had drawn me to him since the days we sat together at the kids table for Thanksgiving, when I knew he would always manage to somehow get us into trouble, with or without my knowledge. And I secretly loved him for that.

As siblings and cousins we had all supported each other as much as possible through the years; even from a distance or when our contact was limited, we knew if we needed we could count on each other.

While Robert had married me several years earlier with his own quirks and history and had ingratiated himself over time with the family, Lauren had married Henry only recently and so remained the only one in our group with whom most of us were not well acquainted; though we had found her friendly and enjoyed her company, we had not yet had a chance to get up close and personal with her. We guessed Lauren had grown up in a somewhat similar family environment, and knew she had been an athlete for some time like the rest of us, but well-groomed and manicured she appeared more polished than we were, and we didn't know how she would fit into our crazy family.

Henry is a recreational outdoorsman, but when he married Lauren it was not for her extensive wilderness experience, and we curiously anticipated how she would take to a week up close and personal with nature. Henry had briefed her as little as possible about the trip so as not to scare her off before they left the comforts of suburbia behind, easing her into the outdoors with a night at the Zion campground on their way to the Grand Canyon, complete, of course, with dinner at the local three-star restaurant. He failed even to advise Lauren that we would be spending eighteen hours a day in our swimsuits, packed into the close quarters of our rafts and scrambling up cliffs, sweating in the stifling heat, and so Lauren had unwittingly packed a *solitary* navy blue tankini bathing suit which she would be all too happy to peel off her body, like a sticky fruit roll from its plastic sheet, and discard disgustingly at the end of our adventure.

"He packed himself three suits, and yet neglected to mention to me that I might want to do the same," Lauren complained sarcastically.

Despite Lauren's lack of wilderness experience, she impressed us with her willingness to adapt to the outdoors and embrace her kooky adopted relatives when on the first day rafting she squatted gamely in the frigid 49 degree water next to me and my sisters alongside the river bank for a "pee stop". Polished hairstyle and manicures aside, this girl had game, and right there, smiling like a schoolgirl while we all balanced in that freezing river current emptying our bladders of the gallons of Gatorade we had consumed in the hot sun, she claimed her own place in the family.

There proved to be no specific routine or schedule on the River, as our days were surrendered to the rhythm of the Canyon's natural motion. Though my diving watch survived the tests of our daily adventures, its demise would have been scarcely mourned, as our days were measured by the sun's passage rather than the rigid movement of the hands on a clock. We embraced days of peaceful floating and raging rapids, meditative hikes to sacred Indian sites and soul-cleansing hidden waterfalls, and lunch stops in scarce shady spots scouted by our experienced guides.

When we tied up the boats along the river's edge for the evening and gathered around in a circle, savoring our gourmet camp dinners, the talk sometimes embraced the philosophical and esoteric but inevitably was punctuated by laughter at sophomoric jokes and family ribbing, with Lauren joining right in. Poking fun at each other amounted to a cherished family sport, made especially enticing by the limitless fodder of material generated over the course of each day in the Grand Canyon.

"Dad, you're going to have to abandon the comb-over or never take your hat off," Heidi teased him mercilessly.

"Same to you, sweetheart," he said, sticking his tongue out at her.

With the river water, heat, and sweat as our daily companions, every day proved to be a bad hair day, and it became difficult to take yourself or anyone else too seriously when you had spent an afternoon bobbing in the slow current of the Little Colorado with a lifejacket upside down around your buttocks and someone else's legs draped over your head, forming a human chain of flotsam in the creation of our very own natural water-park ride. Lauren folded seamlessly into the mix, her easygoing attitude and ability to enjoy life's moments becoming a welcome added dimension to our family.

"You guys are crazy," I heard her say repeatedly in an appreciative, disbelieving sort of way. And nobody could argue. We bonded together as a group with an easy sense of camaraderie, fostered by our isolation from the continuous motion of our daily lives back home, depending on each other minute by minute for survival as well as good conversation.

Admittedly, however, though we suffered our share of injuries and mishaps, our survival never remained in serious doubt. My older sister, Marlene, did emerge from the other side of a bouncing rapid on our fourth day with a nasty bruised elbow that had to be wrapped tightly in bandages, and there were a few risky bouts with dehydration, but my mother proved to be the only rafter who fell out of the boat unintentionally all week. Her tumble into the chilly waters could hardly be considered life threatening, though, as she managed to accomplish this feat while we were floating lazily through a serene section of smooth water. Her fall provided instead another source of comic relief, as she surfaced bobbing alongside the raft in her life jacket and laughing at her own predicament.

"Mom, what are you doing, are you all right?" I asked.

"I'm o.k.! Just help me back in the raft, and John you can reach for your own Gatorade next time!" she barked at my father good-naturedly (well, sort of).

We each in turn stumbled into memorable moments over the course of the week, gathering them like shells at the beach to be turned over and massaged repeatedly. As we floated deeper through geologic time, the beauty of the Grand Canyon revealed itself in the ancient native handprints on canyon walls, the warm turquoise waters of the Little Colorado, the bright green ferns clinging to the damp spaces surrounding a secret waterfall, the thousands of stars shining brightly above us in a nightly tapestry, and the soft light infiltrating the rugged landscape at sunrise.

The deepening of friendships and family ties added to the beauty of the experience, including a developing connection with Henry and Lauren.

I quickly came to appreciate Lauren's sense of humor and storytelling talent, including her engaging tales of Henry's college escapades. And I enjoyed our candid private conversations, responding to their whispered inquiries about babies and apprehension about evolving from a couple to a family. Robert and I were thrilled to hear that they were considering parenthood, and shared our enthusiasm for our three little ones, though I suggested that the ten days of reprieve to raft the Colorado proved to be a welcome break from our pressing duties as parents.

"It's great, but sometimes it can be overwhelming," I admitted.

"So does having children really change everything?" Henry asked somewhat apprehensively.

"Yes, having children changes your life. But in a good way," I answered. I assured them that becoming a family is a wonderful, positive transformation that not only changes your day-to-day schedule and priorities but your fundamental outlook on life as well.

I failed to grow up with mothering tendencies. I had never been a natural second mother to my sister, Heidi, five years younger, or a sought out babysitter for the younger children in the neighborhood. I reluctantly watched Heidi occasionally when my Mom needed to run out on errands, and my babysitting career was limited to a handful of jobs during which I counted the minutes going by, impatient to get back home to a beloved book or tree climbing adventure in the back yard. An independent tomboy at heart, as a child I found myself more comfortable challenging the boys to physical feats than engaging in role-playing with a bunch of dolls, and in college nobody would have mistaken me for one of those girls itching to settle down with a family. Even Robert will admit that when we married he was concerned about whether I would be interested in becoming a mother at all. And, yet, now at thirty-five I found myself happily married with three beautiful children.

"Children are a cherished built-in reminder to live in the moment and not to take yourself or your problems too seriously," I told Henry and Lauren. It is true that a child's laughter has the power to ease the sting of failure or tragedy, and without children I would not smile or giggle or marvel as much, or love as selflessly or fully.

Our shared adventures on the Colorado River, experienced against a backdrop of constant togetherness, bonded us all more closely, and, inspired to reflect amidst the awesome natural environment surrounding us, we thoughtfully considered the fragile gifts of life and family.

Two months later my mom called to tell me that doctors had diagnosed Lauren with cervical cancer. She would require surgery and an intense course of radiation to save her life.

I found out that Lauren had received an initial irregular Pap smear result several months earlier in February, which doctors confirmed again in June after our rafting trip, and that August they diagnosed her with a rare and aggressive form of cervical cancer. Standard treatment would normally have been a total hysterectomy, but instead, Lauren became one of the first patients with this form of cancer to undergo a partial hysterectomy, removing the cervix but leaving the uterus intact.

Unfortunately, though the innovative surgery they performed that October proved successful, she still required intense radiation to ensure the thorough completion of her treatment; radiation which would render her uterus inhospitable. Lauren and Henry kept most of the details private as she attempted to adjust to this new vision of her life which no longer included the possibility of the joy and wonder of pregnancy.

Bitterly disappointed for my cousin, I questioned the sense of fairness in the failure of Lauren's health. Dad had always lectured me, no matter how many times I vehemently railed against it, that *life is not fair*. I could never stand the seeming inequities, mundane or otherwise. ("It's not fair Marlene gets to stay up later......It's not fair Chris gets a bigger piece of cake.") Though I understand now the truth behind Dad's piece of wisdom, I still have trouble accepting its consequences.

Lauren decided in the midst of this bewildering chaos that she would focus more intently on her work, replacing her dreams of a family with renewed career aspirations. Her reaction, while logical, must have felt empty and forced when just a few months earlier on the Colorado she and Henry had shared quietly with me and Robert their wish to begin exploring a path toward parenthood. Unfortunately, they had become statistics of infertility, a condition which dashes the hopes of about fifteen percent of all couples trying to conceive a child.

We all held our breath while we waited for Lauren's body to respond to the cancer treatment. I could only imagine how Henry felt while we prayed for her quick recovery. Henry does not like to indulge events outside of his control, meticulously planning and organizing all aspects of his life, and yet he found himself powerless against Lauren's cancer. I envisioned him researching every aspect of cervical cancer and its treatment in an attempt to dominate this unseen foe.

Though I felt more deeply reconnected to my cousin after our Grand Canyon adventure and I had come to appreciate his fondness for Lauren, I did not think it quite my place (being an intermittent presence in their lives) to inquire directly after Lauren's health or attempt to offer solace. I wanted to, though. I wanted to find just the right words to ease Henry's despair, and to find a meaningful, unobtrusive way to be helpful, to reach back to the past and hold my hand out to the wild-haired boy who had colored my childhood. Without a magic wand to wave away their fear, though, I kept my concern to myself as I waited for news to come through the family.

While Lauren would no longer be able to carry a child, I learned from my Mom through my Aunt Pam that doctors had harvested a record-breaking bounty of 40 eggs from Lauren's hormone-stimulated ovaries before radiation destroyed them. Thankfully, Lauren's astute oncologist had offered Lauren the opportunity to protect her reproductive future by arranging a visit with a fertility doctor to for an egg retrieval procedure. Though more concerned about cancer taking her life, Lauren, on her doctor's advice, took advantage of the small window of opportunity to harvest her eggs, treating it like a side project before starting radiation and getting back to the business of ridding cancer from her body.

At least, I thought, having suddenly and cruelly learned that she had a life-threatening disease and would never carry a child herself, Lauren could hold onto the hope that those eggs, harvested before cancer treatment rudely intruded upon her body, could eventually give her and Henry a child of their own (if she beat the cancer). I prayed for her survival and cheered inside for the possible realization of that hope that they had shared quietly on the River, unable myself to fathom and unwilling to imagine what life would be without my children.

Thirty of the harvested eggs were fit to be fertilized with sperm from Henry through the in-vitro fertilization process, resulting within a couple of days in the successful development of 18 tiny embryos, frozen in storage. By virtue of recent mind boggling scientific advances, the hope existed that one day the opportunity would be there for at least one of those frozen gems to develop into the child they longed to welcome into this world.

From the scare of death had emerged the hopeful promise of new life.

That fundamental wish, though, would now require a relatively unusual set of circumstances to grant it possibility. To pursue having their own biological child, Henry and Lauren would be dependent on a surrogate mother willing to take on the awesome responsibility of carrying their baby for them. Though they also considered the option of adopting, with in-vitro they were given the chance at fulfilling the promise of life to a baby they had created together.

December had arrived when I learned these details; Lauren had thankfully responded well to treatment after several rounds of radiation, and my thoughts turned to their hopes for a child. Curious about Henry and Lauren's options, I found myself gathering information from dozens of informative websites delivering details on infertility, in-vitro fertilization and surrogacy. Typically, I discovered, couples seeking the services of a surrogate have suffered through years of infertility treatments and heartache, and settle on surrogacy as an option only after exhausting thousands and thousands of dollars on other treatments; treatments which had ended in cruel failures and broken promises. Sympathizing with the devastating consequences of infertility, the surrogacy solution fascinated me.

I spent one very late night huddled in the dark in my oldest daughter's room Googling surrogacy feverishly at the computer keyboard on her desk, surfing as many sites and consuming as much information about hormone protocols, embryo transfers, psychological evaluations, and legal procedures as I could find.

But it was the personal stories I read and reread that surrogates and new and intended parents shared online that inevitably captivated my attention and touched me deeply. These personal stories of surrogacy tugged at my heart with their emotional descriptions of desperate parents touched deeply by the generosity of their surrogates, the special bonds that connected them, and the overwhelming joy they shared when a surrogate delivered a baby into their grateful, waiting arms.

I sat there alone in the dark, the computer screen glowing in front of me, with tears slipping down my cheeks.

After I reluctantly closed out of the last site and shut down the computer to crawl into bed in the wee hours of the morning, I remained wide awake, buzzing with emotional adrenaline from my virtual ride through the landscape of surrogacy. Laying there under the covers in the surrounding quiet of the night, my thoughts narrowed in on the unfolding realization of possibility. The unformed, unrecognized, unadmitted thought that had lain in wait even before I began my research on surrogacy began to take on defined shape and weight.

Maybe, just maybe, I could be the one to help Henry and Lauren realize their dream of a family, to bless them with the wonders of parenthood through surrogacy, to give them the joy of a house filled with laughter and lighthearted chaos. Maybe it could be me who gave them all that.

Could I do it though? Could I carry their baby inside me for nine months and then hand it over to them? What would that feel like? You read about other people in the newspaper who are dedicating their lives selflessly to improving the lives of others, people who really believe the noble, but what I sometimes skeptically considered rather trite, call to action to *make the world a better place.* I do not identify myself as one of those altruistic yahoos with boundless energy, commitment, and goodwill who is able to single handedly mobilize people and resources to turn around the fortunes of the less fortunate by sheer will. Thank God for them, but they intimidate me. Maybe though, I thought, if I were a surrogate, I could make the world a better place for my cousin, and helping out in that one little corner might help make the world just a little bit better off in the end. A kind of pay it forward effect.

Did I see myself as the type of person capable of giving generously in that way to someone else, without any expectation? Is that who I am?

Though I already volunteered my time and energy in other ways, surrogacy would require a deeper commitment to giving, but the bottom line was why not? Why not me? The bold outline of my life's path had generally continued along a consistent, established degree of longitude, but I believe it is those side trails which meander back to the main thoroughfare that add meaning and depth to life. Choosing to be a surrogate would no doubt offer the kind of enrichment that ultimately makes the journey along the main road infinitely more rewarding. I had many times experienced the simple joys of giving, but considering surrogacy constituted the first time I had offered to give of myself so fully without the pressure of a nagging sense of responsibility. And though I expected nothing tangible in return, I quickly learned that just by selflessly giving my consideration to the idea, I had already freed myself for greater personal fulfillment.

Henry and I had been close growing up, living only a few miles apart as small children, always reconnecting easily and happily after any absences, as cousins often do. We spent countless weekends together with boisterous family ski trips to Squaw Valley, tree-climbing escapades, never-ending games of hide and seek, and the infamous raucous bed-jumping which ended one night with a trip to the emergency room when my two front teeth broke skin on Henry's forehead.

When we became teenagers, though, Henry's family moved, and we neglected to see much of each other outside of family celebrations. Our lives headed off in different directions, and, in fact, when Henry married Lauren after college, I failed even to make their wedding, attending instead as a bridesmaid in the wedding of a college friend on the other side of the country that same day.

I still appreciated, though, an unwavering, though fainter and less immediate, connection to him, and the River trip had reconnected us with the past as well as traced a path toward a possible future. Now I found myself yearning to lend Henry my hand; the opportunity to help him in such a uniquely special way thrilled me.

I had grown up coveting the idea that I might be special, as I would guess many kids do, but I learned reluctantly over the years that though in truth I might have been unique, I could not claim to be exceptional. I achieved some notable goals in my early years, earning my way into Stanford and reaching high levels of gymnastics, but I discovered along the way that I will always be surrounded by people who are more intelligent, more accomplished, more talented, and more special.

When I reached fifteen years old, my grandmother, MuMu (Justine), treated me to a jam-packed week of New York City culture, including an enchanted late evening at the Café Carlyle with Bobby Short and a whirlwind feast of opera, ballet and symphony performances. One afternoon we visited an elderly Princeton professor, a friend of my grandmother's, and the woman engaged me in a fervent conversation about the state of the present and the future of the United States. When my grandmother and I left later in the afternoon, the retired professor approached me with her hands held out to grasp mine and thanked me for giving her hope for the future, relieved to be reassured that all that she held to be important and meaningful would not be lost in the coming generations.

When she gave me her hands she alternately gave me a burden and a purpose. On occasion I find myself drifting back to the indelible impression she left on my conscience that afternoon, and it serves to guide my direction in the present. If an accomplished elderly woman with all of life's experience and wisdom found something in me that restored in her a sense of confidence for the future, then was it not my duty, my obligation to do something incredible with my life? But what would that be, how would I find it and would I be capable? Could I be worthy of her faith in me?

I never won an Olympic medal or discovered the AIDS vaccine, but I heard her encouragement in my head as I considered the prospect of surrogacy. I did not mistakenly believe that becoming a surrogate represented my purpose in life or that making that choice would help solve the world's problems, but it would be a step, a choice to honor her faith in me and mine in myself that I could continue to reach for the extraordinary.

Although I guessed I probably represented the only relative of Henry and Lauren's who would be realistically capable and willing to act as a surrogate mother, I did not feel an obligation but rather sensed a calling to take that journey. Circumstances had created an opportunity, and the path I would choose to follow slowly appeared clearer ahead of me. I had not yet dived in and embraced surrogacy fully, but I felt prepared to take the first steps along a trail that headed in that direction.

The rush of chatter in my head subsided as I settled in to sleep that night, replaced with a clear picture that made me smile with secret pleasure. I knew now with certainty that I wanted to embark on that adventure with my cousin, to give him the option of walking down the path of surrogacy side by side someone with whom he already enjoyed a comfortable relationship and a shared history. I wished to be Henry and Lauren's surrogate. Me. The next evening I approached Robert cautiously.

"I have been researching surrogacy on the Internet, and I think I would really like to consider carrying Henry and Lauren's baby for them," I confessed cautiously. Raising his eyebrows in surprise and momentarily struck speechless, Robert recovered quickly.

"I think it's an absolutely inspired idea. And I want to support you," he encouraged me.

"But, well, how does that work and what does that mean exactly?"

he asked tentatively. I outlined for him the basics of the surrogacy process that I had researched online.

"What are the risks to you?" he asked, concerned for my health and keen to protect me. "How much more are they than a normal pregnancy?" he wanted to know.

"Other than the hormone shots and the transfer procedure, the medical risks are pretty much the same, unless I become pregnant with twins and then you have the increased risk of carrying multiples. But I'm not really worried about any of that," I answered.

"Of course, it's a no-brainer for **me** to offer up **your** body to carry the baby," he joked, "but as long as the risks aren't too big, you can count me in," he agreed readily.

Relieved, I gratefully accepted his blessing. Robert would be my partner on this quest, his emotional and logistical support would be crucial to me every step of the way, and without his commitment, the surrogacy could have jeopardized the stability of our relationship. Robert, though, is the kind of person who is always looking for ways to help others, friends and strangers alike, and frustrated by his inability to help Henry and Lauren with their situation, he looked forward to this chance to give them hope. He wanted details about what exactly we would be agreeing to before finalizing such a momentous decision, but there proved no need to talk him into it. He loved the idea.

We would be traveling up to the San Francisco Bay Area to celebrate Christmas with Henry and Lauren at my parents' house in a few weeks, and I decided to approach them then with my idea, my offer to carry a child for them.

And so as Christmas approached, underlying my frantic efforts to shop, wrap and decorate, I suffered a twinge of anxiety about gathering together with family to share in the joy of the season. Unaware of how far along Henry and Lauren had progressed in pursuing the option of surrogacy, I guessed that they were still understandably focused primarily on Lauren's fight for health and recovery from cancer. The diagnosis had devastated them. And Lauren, after all, would need some time and space to mourn the loss of her ability to carry a pregnancy before she would be ready to consider someone else carrying a child for her.

I feared, also, that my offer would not only be premature but presumptuous. Would they even want me to carry their baby? Though confident they would not doubt me on the issue of responsibility, I remained unsure they would feel comfortable selecting me to embark with on such a personal voyage. And what words would be appropriate for me to extend such an offer, I wondered?

A few weeks later at my parents' house, as the Christmas evening wound down like the slow deflation of a leaky balloon, I worked up the nerve to approach Henry and Lauren about surrogacy. With such a large family group, it proved nearly impossible to find time one-on-one with anyone, so I rushed in when I discovered an opportunity to speak alone to Lauren, cornering her at the top of the stairs as she searched for her coat to leave.

"Lauren, I have heard that you are unable to carry a baby now, and I am so sorry, but I understand that you have embryos frozen in storage, and I wanted to offer myself to be a surrogate for you if you and Henry choose to take that route," I sputtered, my words tumbling out in a jumbled and breathless fashion into the space between us, looking for somewhere safe to stick.

Lauren appeared somewhat taken aback by my offer and too paralyzed by her surprise to respond beyond a few mumbled words. "Wow. Thank you," she answered back as she fumbled self-consciously with her coat.

I worried in the heavy quiet of the moment that perhaps I had overstepped, that maybe my offer had not been such a brilliant idea after all, that Lauren would not be particularly thrilled with the idea of me carrying her child. I gave her a chance to recover while I filled the pause with my nervous chatter, my anticipation wilting slowly under the lack of an enthusiastic response.

"Just get back to me after you and Henry both have taken some time to think it through," I continued uncertainly.

"I will understand completely if you decide to go through an agency instead. Don't worry about that," I added quickly, in an attempt to give her a graceful out, as the rest of the family drifted toward us to gather their coats and call it a night, cutting our conversation short.

I thought it might be more difficult for Lauren in some ways to rely on me to carry her child, since I claimed status as her husband's cousin and was a family member to her only by marriage. I could not profess to be someone with whom she grew up and shared her deepest secrets, and perhaps it might have been easier for her to partner with a neutral party. There are several reputable surrogacy agencies that specialize in finding and matching caring, reliable surrogates with hopeful infertile couples like Henry and Lauren. I hoped, though, that Lauren felt our connection on the Grand Canyon trip had created enough of a beginning for her to be comfortable with seriously considering my offer to take the intimate journey of surrogacy together. But in all honesty I worried too about the inevitable complexity and potential awkwardness of sharing such a private experience with her, with Henry, with someone other than my husband.

Without an ideal opportunity to speak to both Henry and Lauren simultaneously that night, I had chosen to approach Lauren first because it was she whom cancer had robbed of the joy of carrying a child, she who should have the first right to choose who would or would not carry a child in her place. I wish, though, that I had been able to observe Henry's reaction to my offer of surrogacy when Lauren revealed it to him later that night. How I would have loved to hide under the Christmas presents in the back seat, privy to his initial response and their discussion on the car ride back to his parents house.

Did they think me crazy or inspired? Were they, as I desperately wished, surprised and excited at being given a chance to hope? Proposing to carry someone else's baby for them may be considered a selfless offer, but that does not mean there is not a wish to share in the joy of the couple trying so hard to create a family. It lies at the core of why women are willing to be surrogates. What a thrill it would be to share in Henry and Lauren's joy and excitement surrounding the anticipation and arrival of a new baby.

Though certain about my desire to help them, it still scared me to think about what I had just offered to undertake and what would happen if they actually said 'yes'. Did I really want to take the risk of changing the status quo? And what if I failed to succeed in fulfilling my promise to make their dreams come true?

Again considering the fragile gifts of life and family for which I had renewed appreciation after our River trip, I allowed myself to surrender to my instinct and my heart, to embrace my proposal to embark on a different kind of family adventure, difficulties notwithstanding, to share a life-touching experience with Henry and Lauren, and to grant them their whispered wish for a child. I slid under the bedcovers later that night feeling relieved and a little vulnerable having shared what I held in my heart, but proud of the courage I had summoned to take a willing step into the unknown.

So what did they think of my offer? Henry would call me a few days later.

january 2000

THE DECISION

Choosing Surrogacy

BACK AT HOME IN SAN DIEGO for the remainder of the Holidays, Robert and I celebrated (perhaps a bit too heavily) the prospect and promise of the Y2K New Year with dear friends. Our computers did not crash that night, but my reputation faltered, as I danced uninhibitedly to '80's high school singles, sporting a loopy style embarrassingly reminiscent of *Seinfeld's* Elaine. Blackmail snapshots from that evening documented my suave dance moves, topped off by a pair of shiny "2000" glasses plastered on my face, glazed eyes peering through the zeros. Thankfully, my friends love me despite my many flaws, and those missteps simply became an enduring source of inside jokes and shared laughter.

There were moments during that New Years week, after spotting a stroller parked on the sidewalk or catching a glimpse of my pregnancy clothes bunched up in a plastic bag in the corner of the closet, when my anchor in the present moment would fade away temporarily and my mind would wander back to my brief conversation with Lauren. *What were they thinking?* I wondered, while I waited for Henry to get in touch with me.

Though unprepared to gear up immediately for another pregnancy,

I had invested quite a bit of thought into preparing myself for the possibility of carrying Henry and Lauren's child for them, and I anxiously anticipated Henry's call. Every time the phone rang my insides wound up a little tighter, like the line tension on a fishing reel just before you cast into unknown waters. I knew I could do it, it felt right, and I wanted the opportunity to be their hero, but I was afraid that though they may have appreciated my offer, they might decide in the end to say no, and I feared that rejection, that failure to be found worthy. In my heart I had already cast out a line toward surrogacy, and if Henry and Lauren chose a different direction, the loss of that opportunity would sadden me dearly. I reminded myself to breathe evenly, to keep my fears in check, when I heard Henry's voice on the other end of the line a few days later.

"Hey, Pam. Lauren told me you guys had an interesting talk after our Christmas dinner; that's a really unbelievable offer you made," he initiated. Lauren, it turned out, had waited out the whole car ride back with his parents from our Christmas dinner without saying a word, so that she could be alone with Henry to share my offer, barely containing her excitement until they were by themselves in their bedroom that night.

"Lauren and I are amazed at your generosity Thank you for even considering it," he added, after a pause, conveying his sincere appreciation with a few more stumbling, heartfelt words.

"Your welcome," I mumbled and then added something equally inadequate.

We both felt a little awkward at first attempting to ease our way into the discussion of surrogacy without any sort of script to follow to play out this conversation. Like tiptoeing into the icy waters of Lake Tahoe together as kids, we started with a series of tentative fits and starts before we found ourselves waist deep looking around unsurely. Forcing ourselves to ignore our discomfort, though, we tentatively explored below the surface and acclimated to our surroundings, treading water for a while before we dove in all the way. Henry tenderly, and with obvious concern for me (or maybe my mental state of health), questioned me first.

"Are you really interested in being our surrogate?" he asked in wonderment.

I sat down deliberately with the phone in one hand, and thoughtfully considered his earnest question before I answered. Henry and Lauren would not wish to set their hearts on my proposal if it proved to be just a temporary whim.

"I am excited about the possibility of carrying a baby for you, but honestly I don't really know what kind of leap it would take to go from a meaningful idea to the day to day reality of surrogacy. I would need more detailed information before I could decide for sure," I admitted to Henry.

Henry and Lauren, I learned, had not yet explored the option of surrogacy, and he agreed that we needed to find out more about the concrete realities of the process before any of us would be able to make an informed decision about pursuing it further. Though we had fumbled our way through the beginnings of the conversation, our discomfort eased when we discussed the specifics of the research and discovery process we would navigate in the coming weeks.

And then our conversation faltered a bit again, as Henry made an attempt to convey his gratitude before hanging up. Clearly, I had touched and overwhelmed him with my offer. How should he thank me for even considering the idea of carrying his child, for offering him a thread of hope?

"I don't know what to say, except, thank you," he finally stammered.

The wavering emotion in his voice, filled with a sense of relief and possibility, touched me more than any words he could have chosen, and I hung up the phone, my mind racing, my heart fluttering with excitement. Would it be possible, could we really make surrogacy work? The line was cast now, the tension released into the waters of the unknown.

Shortly thereafter, following Lauren's last radiation treatment in January, the doctors pronounced her cancer in remission. She had won the main battle, emerging cancer-free, and we all sighed with relief, our family bonds growing tentatively stronger.

Lauren, however, overwhelmed with what she had just gone through and still in shock with a lot to sort out emotionally in dealing with her cancer, felt frozen and unable to move forward. Encouraged by her father, though, to move on beyond her illness, she focused on the possibility of surrogacy to help her to regain her balance and the sense of freedom to look forward.

A few weeks after her treatment ended, she and Henry sent me a folder full of information and magazine articles on surrogacy, as well as their synopsis of what would be required to move ahead, including specifically the details and risks of the process itself. Their research served as my first personal encounter with Henry's highly developed organizational skills (some people might call him anal) and propensity for planning. Though I teased him, I welcomed gratefully the sense of security created by his thoroughness. We agreed to take some time to digest the materials and continue researching before we came to any conclusions about whether or not to move forward together.

"Selfishly there is nothing we would like more than to have you as our surrogate," Henry and Lauren opened in their letter to me detailing the process.

And while I carefully read through their research on the medical, legal, psychological, and financial hurdles of surrogacy over the next few pages, I had trouble focusing on anything beyond those first few heartfelt words of approval. There in black and white I finally found confirmation that my offer had been received enthusiastically, and that they would welcome the opportunity to take the journey of surrogacy with me! Their endorsement replaced my uncertainty and insecurity with a rush of excitement and relief. The words of my offer no longer floated out in space, but had indeed found somewhere safe to land and stick. They wanted to choose me, to pick me to play in the game.

"We are grateful and touched.........that you would even consider assisting us in starting a family," they wrote, closing their letter with a warm thank you.

Indeed, they had found me worthy after all, and the thrill of acceptance buoyed me until I felt like a helium balloon in the Macy's Thanksgiving Day Parade, with the strings of reality barely keeping my feet on the ground. While I knew intellectually that there remained quite a bit more researching and analyzing to conduct before making a final decision, emotionally I found it difficult to refrain from taking their hands gently in mine and saying, "Yes! Let's do it; onward and upward!"

As I read through the articles about other surrogates, analyzed the statistics regarding surrogacy success rates, and scrutinized the fertility clinic information detailing the hurdles I would need to leap and the sacrifices I would need to make, I found myself thinking more about Henry and Lauren than myself. This was not really about *me*.

Yes, there would be sacrifices on my part for more than a year at least, but, if given my family genetics and barring any unforeseen disaster I realistically could look forward to 90-plus years to live, what would one single year mean really in the grand scheme of things. And, quite honestly, if I were to have my life cut short by some freakish disaster, would I regret the "loss" of that time?

Time for a reality check: Imagining my spirit hovering above my ashes scattered to the winds on some coastal hilltop, I was certain my regrets would be limited to any time I had wasted needlessly worrying, hurrying, and scrubbing clean the darn toilet bowl. For me and my family surrogacy would require some temporary changes, for Henry and Lauren it offered the possibility of the most dramatic change in their lives. And for their baby out there waiting to be born it represented the chance of a lifetime. Literally.

By April we had all engaged in our own share of soul searching and informational discovery regarding moving forward together with surrogacy, and Lauren and Henry had been able to pause for a couple of months to catch their breath after several intense months of anguish and upheaval from Lauren's battle with cancer.

On Easter weekend they drove down from Los Angeles to join us for a day of egg coloring and repeated egg hunting in the back yard with Kellie (6), Duncan (5) and Lise (2 ½). My children's enthusiasm for finding bright hidden treats among the branches of apricot trees and the coils of the garden hose proved endless, and was only outweighed by my cousin's enthusiasm in searching for ever more creative hiding places to test their hunting skills. The kids delighted in the attention from Henry and Lauren that afternoon, and their mounds of brilliant smiles and giggles matched the pile of bright eggs we had colored that morning. While we shared that joyful day, I sensed my cousin's unspoken vision of a future full of Easter egg hunts and family celebrations in his backyard with his own little ones.

After the kids had been tucked into bed that evening, Robert and I sat down with Henry and Lauren to candidly discuss our thoughts and feelings about embarking together on a voyage of surrogacy. Nervous laughter punctuated our cautious excitement as we poked and prodded each other gently like thorough physicians, probing the health and viability of such an arrangement.

"Do you think this is something you really want to do?" they asked anxiously, seemingly sensitive about overstepping boundaries and asking a cousin to sacrifice too much.

"Yes! I really want to do this for you." I responded fervently.

"Are you both comfortable with the idea of me carrying your baby?" I asked tentatively.

"Yes, absolutely!" they both agreed wholeheartedly, more at ease embarking on a surrogacy journey with family, where there would perhaps be fewer variables beyond their knowledge or control.

I noticed, though, that Henry and Lauren seemed a little less excited and a little more cautious than Robert and me about the idea of surrogacy. But, I thought, understandably so, since the stakes would be unimaginably high for them. Truthfully, I wanted them to be on-the-edge-of-their-seats excited to validate and justify my generous offer, but at the same time I understood that they might feel the need to guard their feelings in order to protect themselves from the vulnerabilities of their position. Realistically, though surrogacy sounded great in concept, it remained disconcertingly possible that at the end of our proposed venture they would come away without holding a child in their arms, and with nothing to show for all our hopes and efforts.

The odds were not in their favor. Henry and Lauren had to commit to surrogacy knowing that there would be no guarantee of success, and it would take time and courage to believe in the possibility of it all. The time sitting together on the couch and facing each other one on one with our hopes and dreams, though, had encouraged all of us to take that leap of faith.

"Let's do it," we agreed.

We chose hope.

There are inevitable risks that accompany any dream, but there is so much sweet possibility, and so we opened our hearts and chose a path that could change all of us.

We chose to dream.

We chose surrogacy.

Reflecting on the reality that the four of us would be joining together to bring a child into the world, we hugged excitedly, marveling at our decision, and for a moment anything seemed possible.

"Are we really going to do this?" Lauren asked hopefully, hardly daring to believe.

It was an intimate moment, not unlike that impulsive flash as a couple when you look into each other's eyes and throw caution to the wind, allowing your love for each other take you where it may, setting events into motion which might make you parents nine months down the road. We all remained fully clothed sitting on that couch, of course, but our thoughts and hopes and desires laid naked before us, as we chose to take those first steps that would give Henry and Lauren the chance at becoming parents. In that instant we all recognized a flash of the kind of faith, trust and love that would be required to take this intimate journey together.

And now that we had summoned the courage to make the fateful decision, immediately, before we had barely had a chance to take a deep breath, some crucial smaller decisions popped up to demand our attention.

Timing presented the most pressing issue at hand: when would we begin?

Multiple evaluations needed to be performed before it would be possible to move forward with embryo transfers, including medical, legal, and psychological examinations. I suggested to Henry and Lauren that if they felt comfortable moving forward quickly, I would just as soon set the process in motion right away.

"Let's get going so we can try to be pregnant by the end of summer," I proposed. (While technically I would be the one physically carrying the pregnancy, truly, we would all be *expecting* a child together.)

I confessed that I would selfishly prefer to be delivering a baby to them before the end of the following summer, because, as vane as it may seem, I was not particularly keen on the idea of showing up barefoot and pregnant with someone else's child at my 15 year college reunion the following October, eighteen months away. I knew that a surrogate pregnancy would inevitably spark a multitude of questions and I preferred not to have that as the focus of my reconnection with old friends. I would not, quite honestly, have even been thrilled to show up visibly carrying my *own* pregnancy for that matter, preferring to be recognized for my youthful fitness rather than for the display of a protruding melon-like belly. A Stanford reunion represented a rare, cherished opportunity to reconnect with that carefree, idealistic young coed I had been 15 years ago, setting aside for a weekend my current all-absorbing occupation as somebody's mommy.

Of course, there are people (who are they exactly?) who say pregnant women are sexy, but I've got to tell you the moments had been few and far between during my previous pregnancies when I felt myself to be anything remotely close to attractive. Maybe it's just that I do not do pregnancy well, but I feel that whole *glowing* thing is way over-idealized, more than likely just a politically correct way for someone to find something kind to say to a woman who has gained a third of her bodyweight, without risking a hormone-induced knee to the groin.

Planning a pregnancy around a due date represented unfamiliar territory for me. My husband and I had never consciously chosen the timing of my previous pregnancies, having discovered that within what seemed like hours of me tossing that month's supply of birth control pills in the wastebasket, he could just breathe on me and I would be pregnant. Now, in order not to disappoint my Human Biology professors at Stanford I will acknowledge I know that scenario is a biological impossibility, but I paused to consider that I had evidently inherited my mother's fertility genes: Pregnancy dominant.

There had proved to be no wait time required after going off of the pill, no need to monitor periods and ovulation, no cause for my husband to start wearing boxer shorts to let loose on his manhood. Those tight BVD's were not an inhibiting factor.

Surrogacy, however, would be a more deliberate approach in which we chose a specific date for embryo transfer. I could appreciate the benefits of this controlled method, even if it lacked the mystery of a typical pregnancy, because it gave the benefit of the illusion that we exercised some kind of control over the outcome of the surrogacy process.

"Why don't we shoot (no pun intended) for an embryo transfer in the summer in a few months," Robert suggested, as we sat there on that couch with Henry and Lauren.

When we had all agreed, Lauren responded with sudden giddy optimism, even though the odds did not appear to be with us given the less than stellar success rates for frozen embryos. We possessed a 15% to 26% chance of succeeding. (That success rate has climbed significantly in the last several years to as high as 35%, though that still means that frozen embryo transfers fail almost two-thirds of the time.)

"I feel good about this, and I see twins!" Lauren shared enthusiastically, hope spreading contagiously within her.

I smiled encouragingly, thrilled to watch her feverish elation embrace the hope of my offer, but I have to admit her response scared me slightly, because I did not feel prepared to carry TWO babies. Henry appeared to be excited too, but somewhat overwhelmed by the whole concept. Granted, it remained a bit odd for him to think about me, his cousin, carrying his child.

Good fodder, though, for a tabloid headline: *Woman Carrying Cousin's Unborn Baby!*

As I closed the door after Henry and Lauren embraced us in a goodbye that evening, I turned to Robert and raised my eyebrows questioningly.

"Well????" I asked, smiling hesitantly. Thrilled they had accepted our offer, now the reality hit.

Robert appeared at least a little nervous about not knowing 100% what we were getting ourselves into, and I could see him thinking *be careful what you ask for, because oh, shit the wheels are turning and I hope we can hang on for this ride!* But still, his eyes dancing, he could not control his boyish excitement.

"This is going to be amazing!" he gushed, his outward enthusiasm helping me to overcome my trepidation in that moment concerning the magnitude of the responsibility I had just undertaken. Yes, the prospect of carrying Henry and Lauren's baby thrilled me, and I wanted so much to be their hero, but the excitement was quickly accompanied by a very real fear of not being able to follow through on my obligation.

"Are you sure?" I questioned.

Not only would I need to jump successfully through all sorts of hoops to prepare myself to carry a child for them, but I began to feel what would come to weigh heavily on me over the next few months as my personal responsibility to deliver the happy ending, literally and figuratively. My cousin, his wife and my husband would all certainly play starring backup roles over the next year or so, but getting down to the nuts and bolts of the situation, it became clear that I remained the one who needed to come through in the clutch.

Could I succeed, could my body succeed, in accepting a foreign embryo, nurturing and growing it, and delivering a healthy infant at the end of nine months? God, I hoped so.

"Yes, I am sure. It will be amazing," Robert whispered reassuringly as he wrapped his arms around me, holding me close.

Before we could initiate medical screenings to determine whether my body presented an optimal environment to nurture foreign embryos or forge a legal contract to cement our decision to pursue surrogacy together, the first step of preparation required all of us to undergo psychological evaluations to determine the viability of a mutual surrogacy relationship.

Choosing the path of surrogacy is an emotional decision for the intended parents and one that deeply impacts the life of the surrogate and her family, and we all agreed that the time with a knowledgeable professional could prove to be invaluable for each of us. Henry and Lauren sought out the services of a family psychologist who specialized in surrogacy, and we scheduled appointments in June for each of us to spend a session with Karen Chernekoff, taking tests, answering questions and sharing our feelings, thoughts, hopes and desires concerning a surrogacy arrangement.

I had never spent time in a therapist's office (my family might argue that such a lapse constituted a gross oversight), and the prospect of an afternoon under the scrutiny of a professional whose job entailed analyzing my thoughts, feelings and responses to determine my emotional stability made me more than a little anxious. Was I normal? Was my desire to become a surrogate healthy?

On the first question, I suppose a reputable professional would not hazard to make a proclamation (though my husband could give you a definitive answer), but the second question was tricky. While some people might argue that merely expressing the desire to become a surrogate clearly labeled me as unhealthy in the mind, the psychologist's job would be to determine if I had approached this unusual arrangement with fully informed consent, including a reasonable set of expectations and motivations, both conscious and unconscious. Would I be mentally stable enough to handle a surrogacy?

On June 20th, Robert and I drove up together to the psychologist's office in Orange County to be formally assessed. Curiously anticipating the afternoon ahead of us, we joked about the possible deficiencies and inadequacies that she might stumble upon in her evaluation of us, as she dredged up the dark secrets of our past.

"She might not even let us back out without a straightjacket," Robert joked.

"Very funny, dear. Speak for yourself," I responded.

Upon arriving, we seated ourselves in her outer office once the receptionist provided us with a sentence completion test, a life events checklist and a personality profile test to complete. These tests would provide the therapist insights into us as individuals and information on how our personalities might match up with the intended parents. The questions probed psychological issues that could surface and our ability to cope in stressful situations, measuring ego strength and self-esteem. After diligently completing the tests like good students, Robert and I joined Karen Chernekoff in her office.

"Come on in. It's so nice to meet you both," she said, as she shook our hands in a warm welcome.

After introducing ourselves and talking in general about surrogacy, Karen questioned us on our relationship as husband and wife and our ties to Henry and Lauren. Robert and I are good friends and partners in life, and I believe we communicated to her the strength of our relationship. Soon enough we felt comfortable sharing our personal thoughts with her on pursuing surrogacy with my cousin and his wife.

"So how do you both anticipate growing your relationship with Henry and Lauren in the midst of a surrogate arrangement?" she asked.

Although, in theory, the focus of a surrogacy is the baby, in reality we were coming to understand that perhaps the most important piece would become our partnership with Henry and Lauren, the intended parents. The circumstances of our proposed surrogacy were different than about 90% of surrogacy cases in which a woman is a surrogate for someone outside of her family, a couple with whom she needs to become acquainted. Henry and I were lucky enough to have already enjoyed a lifelong, comfortable and trusting friendship, and we had established a relationship with Lauren as well, but Karen encouraged us to think about how we would like to see that friendship develop further in the context of the surrogacy.

Though Lauren and I felt at ease with each other, I remained concerned that it might be awkward for her to embrace the idea of me, her husband's cousin, carrying their child.

"I hope my friendship with Lauren will continue to develop, and that we can share in the pregnancy together. I want her to be able to experience vicariously, in any way remotely possible, the joy of carrying a child," I answered Karen.

For his part, Robert viewed the surrogacy as a long-term loan of me to Lauren for the better part of a year or so, not expecting to be included much in the loop with her individually during the surrogacy.

"I do anticipate, though, opportunities for all four of us to spend time together," Robert admitted, hoping as couples we would bond together in mutual support and understanding of a shared goal.

My vision of the ideal surrogacy also included considerable meaningful interaction, working together with Henry and Lauren to create a relationship where we could share our wishes and concerns in a safe environment of mutual support and open communication. My personal fulfillment would come from observing their hope and joy in our quest firsthand.

"I wish for Lauren and Henry to be involved as much as possible along each step of the way, including attending as many doctors' appointments as possible and visiting us to experience my belly growing with their child inside," I added. In other words I wanted them to commit to this pregnancy as their own, rather than each of us carrying on separately in sterile parallel pathways before briefly passing in the night in the hospital when the baby is born.

"Their expressions of appreciation for my efforts to turn their dream of a family into a reality will be a key ingredient in making the journey worthwhile for me," I admitted. I worried that such a thought sounded selfish, but I felt relieved when Karen validated the importance of those wishes in her thoughtful response, rather than psychoanalyzing them as some desperate subconscious call for attention or sign of crazy mental deficiency.

Karen suggested, too, that because ours would be a family surrogacy instead of the more typical surrogate relationship between unfamiliar couples, it would behoove us to come to an understanding on our desired involvement of the rest of the relatives.

"My concern is that though family surrogacy cases can be wonderful opportunities for family bonding, they are actually more likely to get complicated and go south because of the inherent familiarity and extended family dynamics," she cautioned.

Where could we find that comfort zone, and what means could we employ to ensure that it would not be breached? I'm sure Henry and Lauren preferred I not share intimate details about their private struggle with infertility any more than I wanted them discussing my uterine cavity or any other aspect of my anatomy with other relatives. I envisioned this adventure we had embarked upon as a sacred, private one in which the interaction with other family members should be by design, by choice, not by intrusion or entitlement. Having said that, in all honesty I found it difficult to imagine anyone in our families intruding upon our privacy; our parents and siblings had demonstrated respect and support for our decision without meddling over the last several months.

After considerable time in the office together, Karen asked to speak individually to first me and then Robert; primarily, I imagine, so that she could gauge whether our joint responses were in line with how we answered as individuals when queried directly. During my time with her she also took the opportunity to ask questions about my relationship with Robert.

"And how do you feel about Robert's ability to support you in a surrogacy arrangement?" she inquired.

At first I acted somewhat defensively, not wanting to betray Robert and being concerned about presenting a united front. As my level of comfort with Karen increased, however, I realized I would be short-changing all of us if I focused on what I thought I should be saying, instead of sharing my true feelings. I needed to be confident in my relationship with my husband, and know that we had entered into this arrangement with all of the right intentions.

"Robert and I understand each other, and I have no doubts about his ability and willingness to be there for me throughout a surrogacy," I assured her truthfully.

And as we talked, I found relief in sharing my feelings about becoming a surrogate with someone who possessed the experience and understanding to respond intelligently and compassionately to the hopes and fears I carried inside.

"I wonder what acting as a surrogate will really feel like," I mused as we wrapped up our session, hoping that surrogacy would turn into the beautiful experience I envisioned. She assured me that with the foundation of a strong relationship and open, honest communication with Henry and Lauren, it could most certainly be an amazing journey.

"The other surrogates I have worked with say it is one of their life's most treasured experiences," she shared.

I blissfully imagined what that would feel like, but in that same moment I worried how we would all respond if the pregnancy did not take, if I failed, if the journey never really had a chance to leave the shore. I retreated from speaking those fateful words out loud, however, choking them back to avoid the image of failing Henry and Lauren, dashing their dreams on the rocks. We would just have to wait and see which way the winds were blowing on that front.

Though I had approached our session with the therapist reluctantly, I left her office with some new answers, insights and appreciation for what I thought might be one of the most meaningful paths I would take in my life.

Karen invited Robert into her office after me, and probed him individually to confirm his support of the surrogate arrangement. While Robert expected his relationship with me to inevitably change over the course of the surrogacy, he told me he had explained to Karen that he looked forward to the surrogacy as an opportunity to strengthen our connection with each other.

"I understand the inconvenience of giving Pam up for a time, but I feel like the sacrifices would pale in comparison to the benefits of helping Henry and Lauren," he said he told her. Robert admitted to her he worried about the possible medical risks of surrogacy, but explained that our research had allowed his analytical mind to weigh the risks against the rewards, and in the end chose to support our decision to go ahead without any real internal conflict.

Karen also questioned Robert about what he thought were my motivations for approaching surrogacy and what his beliefs were about my ability to handle it gracefully while maintaining my emotional well-being. Without sharing the specific details of his private conversation with the psychologist, Robert assured me of his support and belief in my motivation and inner strength. It pleased me that he too had benefited from the opportunity to speak his thoughts and concerns and gain insights from a knowledgeable and compassionate third party.

On the car ride home from Laguna that evening we both agreed that the therapy session had proved worthwhile, more so than we had anticipated. The time with Karen had encouraged us to talk openly with each other about our thoughts, concerns and wishes for surrogacy, and to consider proactively what we hoped to gain from the experience, particularly the shape of our relationship with Henry and Lauren.

I grew into the surrogacy more comfortably that day; it no longer hung on me so much like a stiff new shirt, the edges had softened and the idea slipped on more easily now.

On June 23rd, Karen recommended in writing to Lauren's fertility specialist (reproductive endocrinologist), Dr. Wilcox, that I continue pursuing surrogacy under his medical direction as the gestational carrier for Henry and Lauren, confident that I had made my decision to become a surrogate mother *"fully informed with regards to the expectations and risks,"* and that I *"willingly desired to pursue surrogacy in an open and respectful relationship with Henry and Lauren."* Karen's endorsement of my ability to successfully follow through on a surrogacy arrangement gave a boost to my confidence in my ability to come through for Henry and Lauren.

I had cleared the first hurdle at least, and I started to feel like maybe I could really make this happen.

THE CHINESE MAFIA

Preparing for Surrogacy

A MONTH LATER, ON JULY 24TH, I climbed aboard the Amtrak Surfliner train, embarking on my first trip from Encinitas to Pasadena for a screening with Dr. Wilcox to begin the medical odyssey in pursuit of our goal. The ride up took a couple of hours and I enjoyed the rare leisure time on my own, away from the organized chaos at home, to catch up on reading the pile of monthly magazines I scarcely ever find the time to enjoy.

Mesmerized by the view of the coastline drifting by through the train window, I allowed my thoughts to drift to my destination and the purpose of today's trip. I shook my head and smiled to myself, as I paused to consider the now very real prospect of becoming a surrogate mom. Though the idea of carrying my cousin's baby still felt a little odd in the face of the natural order of things, at the same time in some paradoxical way, it felt quite right too; so right to give my cousin, Henry, hope for his own family.

For the entire ride up to Los Angeles, my thoughts and emotions were racing unchecked, like the train wheels on that track. Honored that Henry and Lauren had considered me worthy enough to be their surrogate, I now found myself stumbling uneasily under the heavy weight of responsibility of successfully bringing a baby into the world for them. Because though I remained hopeful about our outcome, so much had to go right to make it possible, and my anxiety increased as the momentum built, not knowing if I would be enough to carry it off. But as I considered fully the prospect of surrogacy, my mind quieted and the fears slowly fell away alongside those railroad tracks, overshadowed by the wondrous possibilities, and the bright promise of an extraordinary journey.

"Thanks so much for making the trip all the way up here. Are you ready for this?" Lauren asked eagerly when she and Henry met me at the train station in downtown Los Angeles.

"Of course! It's great to see you guys," I answered, though my apprehension started creeping back as I thought about submitting myself to a medical evaluation. Despite my general good health, I found myself worried about passing what I expected to be a thorough and unforgiving medical review, afraid that my body might betray me under intense scrutiny with its hidden secrets. I worried again about disappointing Henry and Lauren, about taking away the hope that I had granted them already.

After a short ride in their car, we arrived at the Huntington Reproductive Center in Pasadena, parked in the building garage, and then checked in at the front desk before we took our seats together in the waiting room.

While we waited to be called in, we chatted self-consciously and eyed the other patients surrounding us busily reading a dichotomous assortment of glamour and fertility publications. It seemed incongruent to be reading glamour magazines at a fertility center, but I suppose those flimsy publications, full of trivial fluff and superfluous gossip, allow us to indulge in a little fantasy to take the edge off of a harsher reality.

Finally, the receptionist called us in, and, catching my first glimpse of the fertility doc as he walked in the door, I smiled inwardly, recalling Lauren's characterization of him as a Doogie Howser look-alike. Just like the teenage doctor of television drama acclaim from the 80's, Dr. Wilcox looked all of about fourteen. Unsure of what to expect from my first visit to a fertility clinic, I had approached our meeting a bit nervously, but once we sat down for a preliminary introduction and discussion, Dr. Wilcox's smile eased the apprehensive tension in my stomach.

"It's so nice to meet you, Pam. I know Henry and Lauren are excited you have offered to be their surrogate. We're just going to take today to run some preliminary tests," Dr. Wilcox explained.

I pride myself on my ability to read a person fairly accurately based on a quick first impression, and I felt confident that I would be comfortable with Dr. Wilcox. Though his youthfulness may have taken me by surprise, his bedside manner and expertise in our first introduction served to erase all of my doubts about his ability to act as nothing but a respected and highly capable party to our pursuit of a successful surrogacy. And, perhaps most importantly, I felt safe with him. I knew right away that he cared about me and that I would be in good hands.

During the visit I submitted to a battery of blood and urine tests. None of them proved to be particularly uncomfortable, but it was, I mused, a rather different way of approaching the sacred goal of pregnancy. And, admittedly, as they poked me again and again, I started feeling less like a special, compassionate individual and more like a used car being checked out by the buyer's reliable mechanic, who had been hired to look under the hood to search for any potential red flags that would impede a smooth operating piece of machinery.

Henry and Lauren had asked to join me at the fertility clinic so that they could offer their support while I submitted to all the screenings, and their presence reassured me not only that they knew and appreciated the sacrifices I was making for them, but also that we were all enrolled in this surrogacy adventure together. Submitting to medical testing essentially for the benefit of someone else while they waited untouched in the reception area proved awkward at first, but I knew that with Henry and Lauren's support, understanding, and willing involvement we could share in as much as possible of the process together. When the doctor and nurses were finished with their examinations, the three of us departed the office together, hopeful now that surrogacy appeared to be a real possibility.

Henry, Lauren and I strolled up and down historic Olvera Street near the train station searching for a place to stop for lunch before I returned to San Diego. Wandering through the colorful outdoor bazaar, I could not help but wonder as I looked into the eyes of passersby, what their reaction would have been had they known the intent of my visit to Los Angeles that day, and I paused to consider the thousands of other secrets that surely walk by me unknown on a daily basis.

Finally settling in for a meal at an authentic Mexican restaurant, we dug into a lunch of burritos and tacos, bantering back and forth lightheartedly, choosing not to delve into the heart of the surrogacy that afternoon, but instead preferring to let it rest on the side while we delighted in the bonus of enjoying each other's company as a byproduct. Truthfully, I found it liberating that not everything we shared needed to focus on the surrogacy. It made the prospect of the next year or so together less daunting, taking some of the pressure and focus off of my ability to come through, and I looked forward optimistically to the continued development of our friendship.

The results of the blood and urine tests would come back within the next few days, determining whether I had passed the preliminary phase of medical evaluation. Among other things, the lab tested my blood for HIV, theoretically grading, in part, my sexual history. Though unconcerned about the results, I still felt a bit awkward submitting my sexual report card to my cousin for his review. I fleetingly envisioned a family conference in my grandfather's den, with Henry surrounded by cousins, aunts, uncles and siblings while I squirmed in my seat, responding to his interrogation of my romantic alliances over the past 20 years. I blinked forcefully to erase that thought.

After returning home to Encinitas, within a couple of days the faxed report indicated that the blood and Pap tests had come back negative for HIV, Hepatitis, syphilis, and other ailments and diseases. No need for a family conference. The urine screen, courtesy of my tango with the pee-in-a-cup routine, had also come back negative for drugs. Those results, spelled out clearly in black and white, provided Henry and Lauren reassurance that I was beginning this surrogacy steeplechase run in optimal physical condition, giving us the best chance at navigating all the obstacles and crossing the finish line successfully in the end.

Though they had chosen me to be their surrogate in part because of their belief that I would be a responsible, dependable partner, I am sure it had not been easy to lay their trust completely in my hands without any direct control over my choices and actions. The drug results served to give them at least some objective evidence justifying their belief that I would be a stable and trustworthy partner on this journey with them.

For my final medical screening visit to Pasadena a couple of weeks later on the morning of August 3rd, Dr. Wilcox performed a uterine survey to determine the acceptability of my uterus for embryo implantation and growth. I had failed to give it much thought before scheduling our appointment, but unfortunately I had traveled up to Pasadena for a uterine evaluation in the midst of my menstrual cycle. (I had managed to suppress that whole junior high sex education class when they had explained that the *uterus* is the place where, uh, *menstruation* takes place.............).

I am not one to chart the course of my cycle in a meticulous monthly calendar (admittedly, I fail to perform anything meticulously), instead I am usually caught off-guard with that recurring womanly joy once my irritability threshold bottoms out and then I am forced to frantically search the bathroom cabinet for some sort, any sort, of feminine protection. As my Mother had advised me when I started menstruating belatedly at fifteen, a period is a *natural, inevitable event,* so I tried not to be too self-conscious, assuring myself that the doctor had surely examined a menstruating surrogate before.

While Henry eagerly escaped to the waiting room, Lauren stayed with me as I lay down on the examining table. Though apprehensive at first, with Lauren's encouragement and Dr. Wilcox's easy manner I soon felt at ease with the survey procedure. Inserting a catheter with a probe on the end into my uterus, Dr. Wilcox watched a monitor as he performed a controlled survey, looking for polyps, adhesions, and anything that may prevent a successful embryo implantation.

"This might be a little uncomfortable. You may feel some cramping," he advised me.

As I lay there, I imagined a miniature, crude robotic form of the Mars Rover crawling around inside me attached to a long, winding cord, shifting gears to climb obstacles, searching the terrain for hidden secrets and hostile pockets of resistance. Because I had shown up in the midst of my menstrual cycle, the *uterine Rover* engaged in a search and destroy mission to remove all blood clots, rendering the survey somewhat painful, but looking on the bright side, essentially bleeding out my period quickly in one fell swoop. While my visits to public rest rooms for the next couple of days would happily no longer require the highly developed ability to conceal a handful of feminine protection materials in my fist, up my sleeve or in the front pocket of my jeans, I would personally not recommend having a uterine survey on a monthly basis to take the place of the more pedestrian, but slightly less radical use of your basic pads and tampons.

Call me old-fashioned.

"Pam, you have a beautiful uterine cavity," Dr. Wilcox said admiringly during the evaluative survey.

Though it had come out sounding like a really bad pick-up line, I forced myself to stifle a giggle because he said it so earnestly. (Should I have been hurt if he just said it had a good personality?) For the record, Dr. Wilcox was happily married; he was simply an exceptional doctor with an odd sense of medical humor and an admirer of the inner workings of the human body. Besides, he probably uses that line on all of his patients. His comment did, however, prompt me to imagine my uterus as a live pulsating sphere scrubbed to a sparkling clean, walls shining with promise, showing off its best side for the good doctor.

We all rejoiced thankfully when Dr. Wilcox decreed that my uterus had passed the test with flying colors; even he appeared to be as genuinely excited as the rest of us. Feeling relieved, proud, and more confident now that the doctor had declared me medically fit for a surrogate pregnancy, I smiled broadly with the knowledge that we had earned a green light to prepare for an embryo transfer.

Medical hurdle cleared.

To celebrate another step closer to surrogacy, Henry escorted us to lunch at a hip sushi restaurant located nearby, tucked in among a block of warehouses surrounded by chain link fences in a rather questionable area of town. He assured me that he had eaten there safely before, but when we parked the car on a nearby street behind a rather dilapidated looking vehicle, none of us were wholly confident that our ride would still be there in one piece when we returned. We hoped for the best, shrugged our shoulders and walked around the corner and in the door of the restaurant.

Sitting down at our table, we eyed the other patrons surrounding us amidst a striking interior display of vibrant colors, harmonious shapes and rich textures in that modern and upscale, yet still understated eatery. Diners sat huddled in private conversations, engaging in group banter and seemingly conscious of being on display, like fish in a koi pond.

As we perused our menus, Henry discreetly pointed out a group of men who he swore were Chinese Mafia, seated at a commanding table in the corner, complete with a *Godfather* in the seat of honor, guards standing at attention at his side. They left shortly after we arrived, dutiful lieutenants adjusting their sunglasses before deftly escorting their royalty away from the table and out the heavy restaurant doors. As we watched them leave, I unconsciously waited for a movie director somewhere to say "Cut!" to end the surreal interlude. Clearly the mystery of L.A. had taken hold of me.

Despite the vague feeling that I did not quite belong in the crowd there, I thoroughly enjoyed the delectable meal set down in front of us. Over lunch Henry and Lauren talked animatedly, obviously delighted about completing another round of tests and moving us closer to our goal, and we bantered about through lunch in an excited buzz as the surrogacy become a bit more of a reality.

"We are getting so close!" Lauren exclaimed hopefully.

I hopped on the train back home that afternoon to my family in Encinitas, pleased with the surrogacy's progression and reveling inwardly at the hope and joy I had brought Henry and Lauren.

Having passed the initial medical screenings and the psychological evaluation, before we could get too excited we needed to navigate the legal steps that would serve a successful surrogate arrangement. Thankfully, California is one of the most progressive states in the United States, which is one of the most progressive countries in the world with regards to surrogacy. People come to California from all over the planet to arrange legally for someone else to carry their child. Many other places consider surrogacy illegal.

It does not surprise me that different countries and cultures across the globe refuse to readily accept surrogacy, as it is a rather far-fetched concept to grasp at first, and butts up against traditional ideas about conception, pregnancy and motherhood. I find it difficult, though, to believe that people around the world find that there is something **wrong**, something that should be deemed illegal, about carrying another couple's baby for them. While I respect that surrogacy is not the right choice for everyone, or the best choice in every circumstance, I believe it serves a special purpose for many couples looking to end a devastating cycle of infertility through a beautiful, giving offer of hope and love.

Henry found an attorney in Beverly Hills who specialized in surrogacy arrangements, and he drew up a preliminary legal contract for all of us to review. Frankly, there's nothing like sixteen pages of legal rhetoric to abruptly yank the spirit from an offer born out of love and hope, and it seemed almost sacrilegious to catch sight of our tender promise to Henry and Lauren captured in the objective reality of legalese.

Seeing those words in print served to make the surrogacy a more tangible reality, though, and all the rules spelled out meticulously in a binding agreement caused me to reflect on the complexity of our undertaking. If I had retained any doubts about my willingness or ability to carry through with my promise, then that document, designed to protect the parties from ending up in a legal battle over the surrogacy (which occurs in about 1% of arrangements), would have scared me into allowing those concerns to take on shape and weight. Instead, however, those pages served as a welcome concrete first step, inviting public recognition of our faith and trust in each other.

As we reviewed the 41 items contained in the contract, we discovered all kinds of complex issues and frightening scenarios which we had not yet paused to seriously consider.

"Well, this is a fun, inspiring read," Robert joked.

While recognizing the legal need for the contract for the business end of our arrangement, Robert felt an underlying sense of its futility in light of our unique family situation. Though the contract brought to light considerations we had not discussed, it failed to change our perspective, and while it hardly left us with a warm fuzzy feeling about the surrogacy, Robert and I kept a sense of humor as we slogged through endless pages of lawyerly prose, reviewing each section in turn, and editing, amending and supplementing when compelled to do so.

The contract began with a list of "Recitals" that addressed the basis upon which the surrogacy was founded and the intentions of all parties, most notably Henry and Lauren's desire to *have a child or children from the embryo(s) belonging to them and to take such child or children into their home to care for, financially provide for and otherwise raise*. While we found that interpretation of our complex, loving offer to be as stale and dry as a leftover piece of toast, it presented an accurate description of the cold, hard facts, and in the middle of all the medical testing, psychological evaluation and legal procedure, it proved to be a good reminder to stay focused on our shared purpose.

Most importantly, the contract pointedly spelled out that Robert and I promised they we had no intention of having a parental relationship with any child born out of the surrogacy arrangement, agreeing that the baby would be *"legally, morally, biologically, ethically and contractually that of the Intended Parents."* I embraced the words in this paragraph as the concrete foundation of our understanding.

Morally and ethically, we had chosen the path of surrogacy in an honest attempt to bring joy to my cousin and his wife, not intending to give them hope and then yank it away against all codes of decent conduct. In fact, I did not worry that I would in any way want to raise the child after it was born, knowing not only that that privilege belonged solely to Henry and Lauren as the parents, but also that Henry and Lauren would be wonderful parents; otherwise, quite frankly, I would never have offered to bring their child into the world for them. Finally, *biologically*, the egg, sperm, resulting embryo, and baby would maintain no genetic connection to me or Robert.

"Can you imagine even thinking about claiming the baby as your own?" I asked Robert, flabbergasted.

"It seems totally ridiculous," Robert agreed.

One of the most adamant recitals in the contract proclaimed, in capital letters, that *"IT IS EXPRESSLY UNDERSTOOD THAT THIS AGREEMENT IN NO WAY CONSTITUTES PAYMENT FOR A CHILD OR RELINQUISHMENT OF A CHILD"*, igniting visions in my head of a back alley deal with cold cash forked over under a solitary dim streetlamp, in exchange for a white wicker baby bassinet spirited away into the night in the backseat of a black Cadillac.

Though in our case I would not be receiving any lump sum to compensate for my surrogate services, it is relevant and true in any gestational surrogacy arrangement that nobody is relinquishing a child. It is impossible to give something up that you could never claim to be yours to begin with. In my case, in very simple terms, I had offered to loan my surrogate uterus for nine months as a gift to my cousin. But even in most cases when there is an exchange of $15,000 to $20,000 or some similar amount, it is for the services, time and sacrifice of the surrogate that the payment is made, not for the child directly.

A large portion of the meat of any surrogacy contract is dedicated to covering related medical issues. One of the most sensitive points delineated in our proposed contract granted the right of decidding to abort or not abort a fetus with abnormalities to the "Intended Parents". While the Roe v. Wade statute grants a woman the right to choose to terminate a pregnancy for any reason, the ruling (established before the availability of gestational surrogacy) understandably assumes that a pregnant woman is the mother of the fetus she carries inside. The statute is described as vital to the preservation of a woman's personal freedom and privacy, but as a gestational surrogate I would strictly be acting as a temporary refuge and an incubator for the fetus, my body allowing it suitable space for growth and development but devoid of any claim on it, so the "personal freedom and privacy" to make a decision about the fetus belonged in the hands of the true mother, Lauren and her husband, Henry. (In another interesting twist on Roe v. Wade, our contract granted the right to choose to terminate a pregnancy to *both* parents, not just the mother.)

And so though it would be an unfortunate and difficult choice to have to make under any circumstances, clearly the right to make the decision whether to abort would lie with Lauren and Henry. On a personal and intellectual level, I accepted without hesitation that Lauren, though cancer might have stripped her of the opportunity to physically carry a pregnancy, together with Henry deserved the right to make decisions about the future of their family just as if Lauren were the one carrying the baby. I trusted my cousin and his wife to consider all the outcomes and implications of such weighty choices in a careful, deliberate manner full of integrity, and while I felt I would likely agree with them on the choices they made, even if I did not I would still understand and respect their prerogative to make those decisions. I knew that on occasion we might disagree with each other over certain aspects of the surrogacy, but I felt confident that we would overcome those disagreements gracefully, without jeopardizing our friendship or the surrogacy.

Also addressed in the legal agreement was the question of potential physical harm to me, the surrogate, while carrying the pregnancy, in which case the power and responsibility to make the decision on whether to abort would be rightly mine so that I could take action regarding my own health and well-being. While I read over this section of the contract, I fervently hoped that none of us would be required to make any of these heart-wrenching decisions; it would be a depressing failure if all the love, time, and energy invested in this adventure concluded with the agonizing decision to end it prematurely, but it presented a possibility we had to be prepared to face.

My sunny picture of surrogacy did not include the need to make a life and death decision.

Yet throughout the contract document we were forced to confront medical risk issues, including death, which may result from medical examinations, embryo implantations, pregnancy, childbirth and postpartum complications. Other than the embryo implantation, which Dr. Wilcox had assured me was a very safe procedure, all of these risks represented the same ones I had embraced with my previous three pregnancies, yet accepting these risks for someone else prompted a bit more hesitation as I read along. Though aware that even in the 21st century it is possible to die in childbirth, I certainly preferred not to think about the consequences of making that ultimate sacrifice for Henry and Lauren. Robert found these risks even more disconcerting.

"I know it's farfetched, but I can all too clearly imagine Henry and Lauren driving away with their new baby, while I am left alone with the kids, grieving for you," he lamented.

And though the legal contract also states it is incumbent upon the intended parents to purchase a life insurance policy on behalf of the surrogate for the surrogate's family, the protection that that legal item afforded hardly offered much comfort when it forced us to consider my death as a possible consequence of surrogacy. Unwilling to make that sacrifice, the possibility scared me, but the likelihood remained dim enough that the fear failed to take hold, and after giving fleeting consideration to a possible outcome we maintained no control over, we chose to simply bury it beneath our optimism where it possessed no means to scare away the hope we had invested in this journey.

In addition to life insurance, a surrogacy legal contract also covers the necessity of medical insurance and outlines the responsibilities of the intended parents to pay all medical bills related to the surrogacy that are not covered by the surrogate's own insurance. In my case, we were pleased to discover that there appeared to be no exclusions in our insurance contract for a surrogate pregnancy.

We joked about the poor reviewer of our medical records who would be scratching his head trying to figure out why we were submitting pregnancy expenses after the insurance company had paid for Robert's vasectomy three years earlier. (The reviewer, the jaded cad, may have incorrectly concluded that I had strayed outside my marriage commitment for a little something on the side, and it probably would have surprised him to learn that I didn't claim to be the mother of this baby either.) There remained no question that Robert's vasectomy had proven medically successful, as the post-procedure sperm count report had indicated a big fat ZERO.

In fact, as a Christmas present that year Robert had presented me in front of my entire family with a little white box wrapped in a bright red bow; inside was a box of blank bullets accompanied by that lab report. Though I do usually appreciate Robert's sense of humor, his clever play on the words *"shooting blanks"* had left me cringing at the inevitable images they prompted of our sex life at the family Christmas dinner table.

"Thanks, honey. Very funny," I had responded sarcastically. That evening I would have unquestionably preferred to open a little blue box (the word Tiffany's imprinted on it) with a white bow and a very different kind of shiny trinket inside.

There remained a couple of other medically related issues addressed in the contract, including my personal favorite: that the surrogate and her husband agree not to obtain any permanent body tattooing or pierce any body part during the term of the agreement. Understandably, I would not want to expose myself to the health risk of contracting a communicable disease, but I enjoyed a good chuckle over the idea of Robert even considering ever piercing or tattooing any body part. He does not even like getting his hand stamped at Disneyland.

The same paragraph also contained a standard feature of any surrogacy agreement which stipulates that the surrogate abstain from any alcoholic beverages (and of course tobacco and drugs of any kind) for the entire course of the surrogacy.

"Would you guys mind, though, if I drank a glass of wine or beer occasionally toward the end of the pregnancy?" I asked Henry and Lauren hesitantly.

Not that I anticipated a weekly bar-hopping escapade with my girlfriends, and if that were the case I would be happy to ride along as the *Designated Driver* every time, but I knew I had occasionally welcomed a glass of wine at the end of a tiring day on my feet toward the end of my previous pregnancies. I felt uncomfortable signing the contract without asking their permission first, because I knew honesty and trust would be the cornerstone of a smooth and mutually satisfying surrogacy relationship.

Henry and Lauren readily granted me the discretion to indulge in an occasional drink, but our discussion clarified for me that if and when we succeeded in achieving a pregnancy, I would always need to give first consideration to their wishes regarding the welfare of the baby. I could no longer hazard to make such choices unilaterally, because while it would be up to me how many trips I made to the midnight taco stand,

Henry and Lauren deserved to be reassured that their baby was growing in a safe, optimal environment.

In fact, I would have to be sure to make every effort to be more vigilant about my health habits with a surrogate pregnancy. Henry and Lauren had unwillingly been forced to give up physical control of a pregnancy, but I would respectfully consider their opinions with regard to those choices that in any way, directly or indirectly, affected the pregnancy. They deserved that privilege, that peace of mind.

I realized then that while it would only be my uterus, my body on temporary lease to Henry and Lauren, my life by extension would undeniably remain on loan as well, since the demands of carrying a child for another couple would inevitably impact my life choices on a daily basis. However, I did not feel constrained by this revelation; in fact, I had understood from the beginning, when I extended my offer to Henry and Lauren to be a surrogate for them, that such a decision would be all-encompassing, requiring me to temporarily place my life on hold and set aside a year or so in which a surrogate pregnancy would take priority over almost everything else. And, actually, there existed a welcome freedom in having a reason, an excuse, to take a temporary time-out from my life to focus on the needs of someone else.

The surrogacy contract also reviewed some financial issues, specifically to ensure the surrogate does not incur any costs related to the pregnancy out of her own pocket, like lost wages. In my case, I work from home part-time and so my hours are flexible and not inordinately demanding. Because my primary job is the care of my three children, the more likely out-of-pocket costs would be expenses associated with child care should I be incapacitated in any way during a pregnancy and unable to attend fully to my daily duties as a chauffeur, nurse, teacher, laundress, cook, maid, etc.

(Oh, darn.)

A maternity clothing allowance included in our contract allowed me the option to enhance or flat out replace my maternity wardrobe without dipping into my own pocket. While I harbored a fairly extensive range of maternity clothes from my three previous pregnancies, I could barely face that garbage bag full of formless, fashion-less, worn-in-if-not-out pregnancy clothes. I thankfully accepted that insightful allowance to purchase a new set of more modern duds, which would allow me to feel as good as possible while I gave up my body to encompass the awkward extension of a growing baby for nine months.

Our legal agreement also included a monthly allowance to cover expenses such as travel to medical appointments, babysitting for the kids during surrogacy-related outings, maternity exercise and education classes, and other miscellaneous needs like take-out food when I was too darn tired to fire up another home cooked meal. Though the expense for these things is not significant, the allowance provided a psychological freedom from worrying about such added costs, preventing the possibility of resenting paying expenses out of pocket on top of agreeing to put my life on hold for a year to be pregnant for someone else.

Instead, the promise of an allowance offered relief. The contract actually encouraged me to take those mommy-to-be exercise classes that are an opportunity for physical well-being and mental escape, as well as gave me the permission to pay someone else to cook dinner sometimes, considerably easing the daily burden of shopping and cooking at the end of the day when all I might want to do is flop down on the couch and cuddle with the kids.

After slogging through the sixteen page swamp of the surrogacy contract, editing and discussing it with Henry and Lauren, and signing and submitting it in duplicate to the attorneys, we finally cleared the initial legal, as well as medical and psychological hurdles. With mind and body declared fit and appropriate legal protections in place, we could now move forward with final medical preparation for what I fervently hoped would be a successful embryo transfer.

In other words, we could finally get started.

september 2000

THE EMBRYO TRANSFER

Business or Pleasure?

OVER THE NEXT COUPLE OF WEEKS I spoke a few times with Henry and Lauren over the phone, and our excitement about the surrogacy grew exponentially as we anticipated the final preparations for the embryo transfer.

Robert and I had decided to disclose the purpose of my trips up to Los Angeles to the kids in simplified terms, like unfolding the plot outline of a children's story. We considered it important to include our children in the surrogacy experience from the very beginning, not only so that there would be no misunderstandings about the pregnancy, but also so that they could share in the joy of giving Henry and Lauren the gift of a family.

"Lauren was sick and her belly doesn't work right, so the doctors are going to put Henry and Lauren's baby inside Mommy's belly to grow it until it's ready to give back to them," we explained to the kids. Not exactly your typical stork story, but the kids quickly grasped at least the basic premise and spirit behind the arrangement, accepting the surrogacy without hesitation or judgment, albeit with some earnest curiosity.

"How will they get the baby inside you?" Kellie asked thought-fully.

"When will it be ready to come out?" Duncan asked curiously.

"Will we get to see it?" Lise asked hopefully.

After we answered all their questions truthfully, in terms they understood, they grew excited with the possibilities, happy to have the chance to be included in our adventure. They were impatient for us to get started on preparation for the embryo transfer, as we all were.

Finally, on August 17th, Robert and I drove up to Pasadena together to meet Henry and Lauren at the fertility clinic. While the three of them attempted to occupy themselves in the clinic's waiting area, Dr. Wilcox conducted an ultrasound to examine my uterine wall thickness, and I donated blood again to test estrogen levels. Thankfully my body appeared to be on track, allaying my unwarranted fears about the possibility of suffering a delay in our timetable for the transfer. In my mind I rationalized that if every step of the journey proceeded smoothly, then we would be set up for success in the end, blessed instead of jinxed, so every little victory that signified our luck still held became critically important to me. I did not want to be responsible for any hiccups in our progress, concerned about how such delays might affect Henry and Lauren's confidence in me and mine in myself.

With the testing completed, Dr. Wilcox sat me down and explained the hormone shot regimen I would be starting up to prepare my body for the embryo transfer and then continuing on for the next twelve weeks. The estrogen shots to thicken the endometrial lining of my uterus would begin immediately with a syringe shot into my buttocks administered every third day, while the progesterone shots to improve the uterus lining and embryo implantation would require a similar daily administration, but would not begin for another 11 days. Additionally, at least for the first six weeks, I would be required to wear an estrogen patch on my belly 24 hours a day to allow estrogen absorption directly into my uterus through my skin, and I would need to take progesterone lozenges daily when I began the progesterone shots. Wow. That's a lot of hormones.

Overwhelmed by a schedule that appeared to require a Blackberry just to manage its intricacies, I felt like a science experiment at the whim of outside influences, unsure of how my body and emotions would respond over the course of the next 12 weeks to a chemical invasion. Would this be like an agonizingly long case of PMS? Or worse?

Dr. Wilcox' nurse met me and Robert in a small examining room to demonstrate and begin the hormone regimen. She stabbed a syringe full of estrogen hormone fluid into my right buttocks, pulling back on the plunger and releasing the contents into my body.

"Massage the fluid in gently to prevent soreness and tough tissue masses which might make later shots more difficult and uncomfortable," she advised matter-of-factly. As I stood there whimpering quietly to myself in recovery, I thought the whole shot regimen thing might regrettably become somewhat of a burden, and I hoped I would not be a baby about it. "Be strong" I told myself, because I feared it would be too easy to become weak and collapse into resentment.

The nurse tore open the package for the estrogen patch and adhered it to my belly, requesting that I change it every day and reapply a new one in approximately the same location. Appearing like a gargantuan band-aid on my midsection, the patch held serious potential as a sexual turn-off, serving to remind and reinforce our imposed prohibition from sexual activity for the next six weeks; more of the doctor's orders.

A few minutes later, I decided that while the shot had proved to be uncomfortable it would not be an unbearable sacrifice, and I felt confident that Robert and I would be able to handle repeating it without too much difficulty. With the hormones now on their way inside my body, it finally felt like we had officially begun the preparation for Henry and Lauren's embryo to be transferred into my uterus. I hoped the estrogen had already started to work its magic to prime me for the *Immaculate Conception,* or "immaculate reception". Technically I suppose the conception had already taken place, and admittedly I felt more like Pittsburgh Steeler Franco Harris receiving a fateful pass than the beneficiary of a miracle of God, though a successful surrogate pregnancy is often considered a miracle of sorts.

The doctors had required Robert to attend the clinic that day as wel, to have his blood tested for HIV and to supply a urine sample for analysis. I think he felt useful that day for the first time in the surrogacy process, happy to make some kind of personal contribution to our joint endeavor beyond his indirect support of me.

But on his way back to the waiting room a nurse approached him for one final test, handing him another cup and pointing to a door at the end of the hall. I observed the hastingly concealed look of embarrassed shock on Robert's face and quickly I realized, much to my surprise, that they required him to submit a sperm donation. Not exactly the kind of *contribution* he had anticipated. Robert walked reluctantly behind the nurse, his shoulders bowed, like a chastened child down the long corridor, and I cringed slightly as he closed the unmarked door behind him resignedly. No matter how discreet the office personnel try to be, you might as well have a big sign on that door that shouts: *Sperm Wanted. Enter and Donate on Command.*

Back in the waiting room, Lauren and I smiled sheepishly in surprise. Henry sat slumped over in his chair, wincing sympathetically for Robert, worried I think in that moment that he was asking too much of us. When Robert stepped back down the hall several minutes later, we eyed him carefully, waiting cautiously for his response.

"Thanks a lot for sabotaging me! You guys could have at least warned me that I would be required to sit in a darkened room with a girlie magazine, coerced into making a donation for the cause," Robert accused us jokingly.

"Robert, I swear I had no idea or I promise I would have warned you," Henry said, shaking his head apologetically as we all got up to leave the clinic together.

"Yeah, yeah, yeah," Robert responded, with an exaggerated eye roll.

In truth, for Robert the request, though surprising, had really not been that big a deal, and we all managed to smile resignedly together in solidarity at just one more unusual experience on this road to surrogacy. We had survived our clinic visit, and so we could look forward to an evening of relaxing and celebrating with Henry and Lauren as our hosts. We drove off together to attend a game at Dodgers Stadium, the kids safe at home in the care of a babysitter for the night so we could enjoy a rare and treasured evening out.

As we parked the car upfront in some VIP spot Henry had secured in advance, I connected those three letters on the placard on top of the car dashboard to my new elevated status as a *very important person* in my cousin's life. I sensed an inconspicuous change in our relationship that evening, as Henry slipped subtly into the role of my caretaker, treating my comfort and well-being as his responsibility and priority. Though I am usually strong and fiercely independent, when I am feeling vulnerable I will surrender to the urge to be protected, and Henry's attention comforted me. At that moment I knew without a doubt that he would watch over me through any difficult moments of surrogacy. I appreciated deeply the security of knowing that he and Lauren would be there with me one hundred percent every step of the way.

While I smiled inwardly at these comforting thoughts, we all followed a path into the ballpark, pulled along with the rest of the crowd, the surrounding scene appearing like a squeaky clean Disney image infused with a rainbow of bright colors. A beaming usher escorted us to our seats directly behind the net at home plate. I mean you cannot get any closer; we were practically on top of the catcher for god sakes. Robert and I are both fans baseball, and though the Dodgers are not our team, we readily appreciated the opportunity to enjoy an evening behind home plate at Dodgers Stadium.

A resident of the Bay Area and San Diego for most of my life, I have to admit I have never claimed to be a Dodgers fan. In fact, as a Giants or Padres fan it is unthinkable to do anything but loathe the Dodgers. Not particularly given to the rivalries of Major League Baseball, though, I found it easy enough to enjoy the game and cheer for a play well done. Lest I offend any Giants or Padres fans, I can assure you I refrained from any outright cheering for the Dodgers. I am not so easily bought with prime seats and free food.

We basked in the game atmosphere and the privilege of the seats we happily occupied, occasionally breaking the rhythm of watching the game to talk excitedly between at-bats about the upcoming embryo transfer in a couple of weeks. We were all optimistic that the hormone shots would accomplish their intended job, and we looked forward eagerly to the embryo transfer scheduled for Labor Day weekend. I enjoyed a magical night sitting there soaking up the excitement of the game, holding close my eager anticipation of the next few weeks and months. We celebrated that night a turning point in the surrogacy for all of us, from a hesitant possibility to the promise of a future.

Back at home, I continued with my estrogen hormone shot regimen to prepare my uterus for the embryo transfer, although my buttocks were beginning to resemble an enlarged pincushion. I quickly determined my inability to administer the injections alone without performing challenging physical and mental gymnastics. Dr. Wilcox' nurse had suggested standing in front of a mirror when I attempted the shots, and while I could see well enough to find the rather large target for the needle plunger, I found it awkward to position the needle in my hand well enough to be able to jab it in properly. More crucially, I struggled to gather up the courage to gouge myself voluntarily. It had seemed so much easier when performing practice injections on an inanimate banana. As a consequence of my failures, the privilege of performing that daily task fell to my reluctant husband.

Robert's history of faintheartedness when circling within ten feet of a needle, as evidenced by the epidural incident with my first delivery, caused me to be a bit hesitant (to say the least) about engaging him in the hormone protocol. I nearly resigned myself to scurrying down the street in my bathrobe every morning, syringe in hand, and knocking on the door of my neighbor, Diane to enlist her expertise as a nurse. Robert, though, for my sake, willed himself into conquering his discomfort with flesh and blood, proving his mettle to my great relief by quickly becoming an expert on hormone injections. I appreciated his efforts greatly, aware that he had never aspired to a career in a medical field. Robert's childhood dreams had been more closely aligned with the practical ingenuity of detective Jim Rockford and the cunning Mac-Gyver, than with a white-coated Marcus Welby, M.D.

We devised a morning routine in the bathroom, prepping for the shots like a methodical surgical team. I prepared the syringes by filling them with the required medication while Robert rinsed off in the shower, and as soon as he had toweled dry I handed them over, finding a soft spot on my hiney that had escaped compromising soreness or irritation from previous shots and pointing to it reluctantly. Robert would eye the target carefully, check that the syringe appeared in proper order, give me a warning like the official at a boxing match, and then quickly plunge in the needle, gently pushing the syringe in and forcing the medicine out and into my body. Withdrawing the needle, he held it up to the light to check that the syringe had released every drop, and when he sealed the used apparatus in a plastic bag to be carefully disposed of later, I massaged the medicine in cautiously to hasten its distribution.

The success of the routine varied each morning. On some occasions I collapsed into self-pity like an injured animal, when the syringe entered a sore spot on my buttocks, wounding me unceremoniously. I would stifle a yelp and grit my teeth during the painful exit of the thick liquid, while Robert cringed apologetically, willing the pain away. On those mornings in a fit of frustration I entertained fleeting second thoughts about this brilliant adventure called surrogacy, but the moment would pass quickly and I would emerge with empathy for my friends who had suffered a similar shot regimen in their own efforts to overcome infertility. Other mornings I would barely feel the pressure of the needle in my flesh, and turning to see when Robert would be delivering the shot, I would find him triumphantly holding up the emptied syringe like the flame of the Statue of Liberty, much to my relief and appreciation.

Alas, any last bit of modesty I had managed to salvage following the compromising indignities of my three previous pregnancies and deliveries had dissolved like an Alka-Seltzer tablet with these new daily intrusions. Surrogacy is not a solitary experience, it is a team sport, and as such it required me to willingly give up my privacy as a means to an end, to include the assistance of my husband, the wishes of my cousin and his wife, the evaluation of my thoughts by a psychologist, the monitoring of my body by a fertility team of professionals. While I did not resent this expansion of my private world, I wished sometimes that I could retreat to my own space by myself, to re-establish some boundaries on the playing field.

On August 28th back in Pasadena at the Huntington Reproductive Center with Lauren, Dr. Wilcox monitored estrogen levels in my blood and examined my uterus by ultrasound for the third time to determine implantation readiness.

"Your body appears to be right on schedule for our Labor Day Weekend embryo transfer date," Dr. Wilcox concluded. At least, thank God, all those intrusive shots had not been in vain; the hormones were working successfully to mimic a traditional conception.

After reviewing with me the instructions for a daily progesterone shot and lozenge to be added to my estrogen regimen (ugh, more shots!), the nurse delivered the first dose of progesterone immediately right there in the clinic. In addition to encouraging the endometrial lining of my uterus to grow and flourish, the progesterone would signal my pituitary gland that no menstrual period should take place. Though not thrilled to have to endure more painful intrusions, I could celebrate that finally, in just a few short days, a group of tiny embryos frozen in storage for the last year would be given the chance to find fertile ground in my hormone-hyped uterus.

A year had passed since doctors had diagnosed Lauren with cancer, eight months since I had offered to be a surrogate for Henry and Lauren, and five months since we had decided to proceed with surrogacy. Hope and determination had carried us through months of treatment and recovery, discussion and evaluation, as well as psychological, medical and legal preparation to get to this point in our journey. Though it had taken time and effort to walk the path of surrogacy, my enthusiasm and dedication had not waned over the preceding months while we navigated the course of obstacles, and I celebrated as we continued to move forward with every fortunate, triumphant step in our goal to reach beyond the world of infertility. My eagerness to bring a child into the world for Henry and Lauren had monopolized my thoughts and attention for weeks and weeks; in the shower, at soccer games, preparing dinner, when my head hit the pillow, and I became impatient to actually start my role as a surrogate mother.

We scheduled babysitting arrangements for the kids for Labor Day weekend well in advance, so that Robert and I could travel up to Pasadena together for the big event. When that first Thursday in September arrived, we packed our weekend bags (including the ever-present syringes and hormones) and embraced the kids in tender hugs goodbye.

"I hope you get a baby, Mommy," Duncan said.

"Good luck!" Kellie said.

And closing the garage door behind us that afternoon, we at last motored down the street toward the freeway to Los Angeles for the much anticipated transfer.

Quiet at first on the ride up in the car, Robert and I were both feeling anxious (anxious-nervous as well as anxious-excited) about the prospect of beginning the journey of a surrogate pregnancy with Henry and Lauren. The stakes were high for all of us.

"I can't believe we're actually doing this. This is your last chance to back out," Robert joked lightly.

"Very funny, honey," I responded, raising my eyebrows in sarcasm.

But the truth was, he was right. This was it. There would be no backing out after I accepted their embryo into my body. Not that I wanted to, nor had I ever seriously reconsidered my offer, but this step made it all of a sudden so real, so present, so NOW. All the preparations we had made and all the steps we had taken on our journey so far had committed me more to our agreement, our relationship, and our partnership. I did not find myself hesitating now, but the idea that we were actually at the critical point of realization still managed to take my breath away.

Recovering from that thought, I talked with Robert about our hopes for a successful transfer and our hopes for ultimately fulfilling this dream for Henry and Lauren. And though excited to begin, we still worried about the unknowns and the possible awkwardness of sharing a pregnancy with another couple. Would we find our way gracefully through the inevitable uncomfortable moments? I wondered again what it would feel like and how it would be different, to carry someone else's baby inside me. And we both mused, if successful, the pregnancy would last nine months, but the influence of that quest to bring a new life into the world would become part of us forever. How would it change our lives, our outlook?

Arriving at the front doors of The Huntington Ritz Carlton that evening, allowing our questions to sink below the surface to linger unanswered, we admired the classic beauty of the hotel and its lush grounds as we stepped outside and into the peaceful surroundings. Henry and Lauren had arranged for our weekend stay at The Ritz Carlton as a gift in appreciation for embarking on this journey with them, providing a blissful environment in which to serve out my prescribed rest and relative inactivity for the 48 hours following the embryo transfer; a minimum security incarceration: Relaxation. Luxury. Escape. Not exactly San Quentin.

Wandering up to the check-in desk in the elegant lobby, we gave the clerk our name to locate our reservation. After welcoming us to the hotel, he inquired politely about our stay, as I am sure he had thousands of times to previous guests.

"Have you arrived for business or pleasure?" the clerk asked matter-of-factly. Robert and I, caught off guard, turned to each other reflexively, hesitantly, unsure of how to answer that seemingly simple question.

"I don't really know how to answer that. A little bit of both or none of either, I guess," Robert replied apologetically after a long pause. Though confused, the concierge hesitated only slightly, recovering his poise quickly without probing us further, and handed over our key with directions to our room. We carried our light luggage to the elevators, exchanging conspiratorial smiles as the doors closed after us.

"That is a very interesting question," Robert mused as we rode up to the 4th floor.

The facts: We had traveled out of town for an embryo transfer attempt in anticipation of becoming a surrogate for my cousin and his wife: *Business or pleasure?* While it represented a legal arrangement, a surrogacy failed to constitute a typical business deal, and though we planned on enjoying the weekend away, and more long-term the prospect of making Henry and Lauren parents, I would not consider undergoing a medical procedure to be a pleasurable experience. The truth is a venture through surrogacy is a little bit business, a whole lot of love, trust and sacrifice, and an abundance of pleasure delivered at the end. *Business or pleasure?* It remained a quirky conundrum that continued to amuse us for the rest of the afternoon.

We admired our deluxe room and walked the grounds that evening after an early dinner in the hotel café, watching a movie in bed before going to sleep for the night. Though anxious about the next day, being the sleep-deprived parents of young children we fell easily into a restful slumber in the luxurious appointments of an overstuffed, oversized Ritz Carlton bed.

Henry and Lauren arrived in a state of excitement the next morning to collect us for the short drive to the fertility clinic, chatting all the while in giddy anticipation, relieved on some subconscious level I think to find that I had not reconsidered my offer at the critical moment.

"Here we go guys!" Lauren squealed, eyeing me hopefully.

I smiled at them from the back seat of their car, quietly contemplating the momentous morning ahead and reveling in their enthusiasm as I grabbed Robert's hand anxiously for support. I felt like a prized protégé being chauffeured to a highly anticipated debut performance, coddled with kid gloves in appreciation, admiration and wonder.

At the fertility clinic I changed out of my clothes and Dr. Wilcox completed a final ultrasound check of my uterus with Henry, Lauren and Robert all in attendance in the examining room. The mood had shifted slightly now, the giddiness retreating to hope and expectation while the reality of the risks and consequences of the embryo transfer faced us squarely on.

My uterus appeared primed and ready after weeks of hormone injections, and Dr. Wilcox gave the final thumbs-up for embryo transfer. Lauren clasped her hands together tensely and Henry wiped his sweaty brow in that chilly sterile room as Dr. Wilcox briefed all four of us again on the details of the procedure.

"I would like, because of their current condition, to transfer all four of the thawed embryos," he informed us firmly in this final moment.

We all balked immediately at Dr. Wilcox's wish to transfer all four embryos, having been under the impression that they would only be transferring two embryos from the straw of four the embryologist had thawed from frozen storage.

Henry and Lauren possessed a total of four separate groups (*straws*) of embryos frozen in storage. With each transfer attempt, one entire straw of embryos is thawed, and each individual embryo is evaluated for its implantation potential. Because after Lauren's cancer radiation treatments doctors could no longer harvest eggs from her to create more embryos, Henry and Lauren had only the four attempts at an embryo transfer, four shots at making their own baby. I fervently hoped that this first attempt would not be a strike, as I knew the pressure would increase exponentially with each failed implantation attempt. However, none of us had initiated this quest prepared to assume the possible consequences of transferring four embryos into me simultaneously.

Robert and I had spoken earlier with Henry and Lauren on at least a couple of different occasions about our concerns regarding carrying more than one baby. While I felt that I could handle carrying twins if that proved to be our fate, I did not feel comfortable about the astronomical risks that accompanied carrying more than two, should more embryos implant successfully. And none of us wanted to face the prospect of what doctors call a "selective reduction", forcing us to choose to eliminate embryos, though we had agreed that reduction would be a possible option with a multiple implantation in order to ensure my safety and that of the pregnancy. Which implanted embryos would you choose to eliminate and how could you ensure that the procedure did not adversely effect the remaining ones? How could you feel good about that? I feared our situation could turn into a risky game. Bottom line: I hoped for a safe hit, a single preferably, not a grand slam.

"I strongly suggest transferring at least three embryos in order to improve our odds of success," Dr. Wilcox gently insisted.

The final decision, though, was ours. As I lay there half-naked on the examining table, the four of us engaged in a flurried discussion of risks and benefits on the number of embryos to be transferred, thankfully coming to a quick and unanimous consensus of three. In the end I believe our decision to transfer the three most promising out of the four embryos satisfied Dr. Wilcox, primarily because the odds on the fourth presented a long shot anyway, as it had failed to progress successfully in dividing during the preceding 48 hour thaw period. I found it infinitely reassuring that morning to observe Henry and Lauren's concern for my well-being as the priority in that earnest exchange, at an instant when all their hopes and emotions remained caught up in those four tiny embryos.

Henry and Lauren bowed out of the room after we had communicated our wishes on the embryo transfer count, squeezing my hand and kissing my forehead supportively as they left to stand by in the clinic's waiting area. Dr. Wilcox called in Dr. Tran, the embryologist, asking him to prepare the embryos for immediate transfer, and Robert and I glanced nervously at each other in anticipation while Dr. Tran exited to another room to meticulously load up a catheter with the three chosen embryos.

"Pam, you'll do great, just think of your uterus like a catcher's mitt," Dr. Wilcox encouraged me, making the last minute preparations. Robert and I smiled at yet another conversational gem of medical insight from Dr. Wilcox, attempting to imagine a baseball glove enveloping the embryos securely in its grasp.

"The embryos are ready for implantation," Dr. Tran called back over the intercom. Dr. Wilcox gave him the green light for transfer.

Ready. Dr. Tran quickly stepped in the door, a masked embryologist carefully cradling the syringe attached to a long, thin catheter in his gloved hands.

"I have here three embryos of Henry and Lauren," Dr. Tran confirmed with Dr. Wilcox, identifying them to ensure the transfer of the correct embryos into the designated uterus. Briefly pausing to consider the consequences of mistakenly carrying the embryos of some other couple, I found it reassuring to know the Huntington Reproductive Center monitored procedure vigilantly. *Set.* Dr. Wilcox spoke reassuringly to me as he assisted Dr. Tran in inserting the catheter through my cervix, releasing its contents into my uterus: *Aim, Fire!*

Within a couple of minutes the doctors completed the procedure and I marveled at the simplicity of the process. Granted, all of the preparations to bring us to this moment had proved anything but simple, but the transfer itself proved to be beautifully uncomplicated. It was not, however, anticlimactic, as life can sometimes be when the build-up for an event is so great and then the event itself passes by unexpectedly quickly and without fanfare. The simplicity of the embryo transfer procedure had in no way diminished its awesome purpose.

Dr. Tran retreated from the room with the empty catheter to return to his laboratory and confirm that he had transferred all three embryos successfully. As we waited, I inhaled purposefully, breathing hope and willing life into my uterus, pleading privately for, well, a miracle: A baby for my cousin, a family.

"The catheter is clear," Dr. Tran radioed back to Dr. Wilcox over the intercom, confirming the completed transfer.

"This whole episode feels like a surreal Saturday Night Live (SNL) skit of a NASA shuttle launch," Robert leaned over and whispered. "Houston, we have clearance. The embryos have lift-off," he mimicked. I smiled in response as I imagined SNL's Dennis Miller ripping off a rapid fire of embryo transfer one-liners over the other end of the intercom, but the intercom speaker remained quiet as Dr. Tran attended to his duties as an embryologist back in the laboratory, devoid of any known aspirations to become a stand-up comedian.

The procedure had proved quick and painless, and Henry and Lauren returned to the room to be with me while I followed the doctor's instructions to remain lying down on the patient table for 30 minutes as the embryos gently settled into place inside my uterus. I imagined three tiny parachutes floating gracefully down underwater to land softly in enveloping uterine tissue. We all remained hopeful, as the four of us crowded together in that examining room waiting for those three little guys (or girls) to grab hold.

"I have a feeling it's going to be twins!" Lauren proclaimed in that moment of giddiness, confident about the success of the transfer. I, on the other hand, weighed down by the enormous pressure of the moment, hesitated to be so quickly optimistic, focusing my energy instead on continuing to silently rally them, any of them, to have the courage and tenacity to hold on to my uterus for dear life. Please.

Shortly, after reviewing once again the continuation of my hormone regimen, Dr. Wilcox released me from the clinic under advisement to keep my feet up as much as possible and avoid any strenuous physical activity over the next 48 hours, advice easily and happily followed in the confines of the Huntington Ritz Carlton.

The four of us returned to the hotel to celebrate the embryo transfer at lunch in the hotel dining room. I felt oddly calm and vulnerable in those first few hours, cautiously restraining myself from engaging with the outside world and allowing my protective instincts to dictate my actions, intent on making prudent choices to ensure the best possible opportunity for the embryos to take hold. Henry and Lauren buzzed with hope at lunch, intoxicated with the idea that their baby had found a home inside my belly. Robert, too, hummed with energy, bursting with the proud news of the transfer until he felt compelled to share our story with the hotel concierge when he requested a stool to keep my feet up, per the doctor's orders.

At lunch, with my feet dutifully raised, the four of us alternately spoke jokingly and earnestly about the transfer procedure, as I carefully guarded the precious package inside of me like a mama bird coddling her eggs. The three of them hovered around me in a protective shield, seemingly ready to leap in front of me to protect my womb from an errant falling chandelier or stray speeding bullet, though I noticed no perceptible California earthquake tremors or Chinese mafia lunching in the dining room with us that day. Henry and Lauren lingered with us over our meal, reluctant to leave me behind with their precious cargo, and then hugged me, *gently*, goodbye as they headed out for their own Labor Day Weekend getaway with friends in Palm Springs.

"You guys enjoy the rest of your stay, and we'll get in touch with you when we get back in town," Henry said.

"We'll be keeping our fingers crossed!" Lauren added.

Back in our hotel room, Robert decided to take advantage of the opportunity to nap uninterrupted by the pitter patter of little feet, and I rode the elevator back down to the lobby, stepping into the hotel spa for a massage which Lauren had scheduled for me as a thoughtful surprise. For the hour that I lay there in the semi-darkness I communicated without interruption with those three floating embryos inside of me, sending out to my belly every ounce of positive energy and encouragement I possessed to assist them in their attempt to find a safe place in my uterus to call home. The massage forced me to relax, successfully serving to ease the tension I carried as a burden of the expectations surrounding that morning's transfer attempt.

Robert and I lounged poolside for the remainder of the afternoon, reading magazines absentmindedly and speaking in whispers about the events of the day, our eyes sparkling with hope like the reflection off the water in that turquoise oasis. Superstitiously, I remained relatively motionless on that chaise lounge, making my best effort not to jostle those three little ones inside me so that nothing would disturb them from settling in comfortably. One of my closest friends, Maureen, took time out of her afternoon and away from her four small children in nearby Los Angeles to visit with me and offer her companionship and encouragement. The heartfelt support and admiration for our endeavor that she shared with me during her brief visit nourished me that afternoon and strengthened my confidence for the anxious hours ahead.

That evening Robert and I ordered room service and watched movies in bed, and I made occasional restrained gleeful forays to the hospitality room to scavenge snacks, shuffling cautiously down the hall. While we lay in bed that night, protectively guarding Henry and Lauren's future, my body tingled with anticipation. Were the embryos taking hold? Would I fulfill my special role as a surrogate mom? Had we succeeded in granting my cousin's wish? My body guarded a secret, and it would be days before I discovered the truth, but I anxiously reveled that night in the wondering as I curled up to fall asleep, emotionally exhausted from the climactic events of the day.

After sleeping in the next morning and then a visit to view the painting masterpieces at the nearby Norton Simon Museum, we checked out of the hotel. A note from Henry and Lauren waited for us at the front desk, wishing us a Happy Labor Day with promises to call when they arrived back in town, and I felt reassured that their thoughts remained with us over the holiday weekend. On the car ride back down to San Diego I sat quietly in an anxious state of awareness, my hands involuntarily drifting toward my belly, until we arrived back home and into a chorus of welcoming shouts from our three children.

"Mommy!" Lise exclaimed, her face lighting up with a smile, glad to have us back home. Not quite three yet, she seemed both relieved and thrilled that we had miraculously returned, secure in the knowledge that now all would be just the way it should be again.

"Is the baby in there now?" Duncan asked curiously, while Kellie

stared hard at my belly, looking for any discernable change in my appearance.

"Well, we hope so, we have to wait a week to find out," I explained.

Over the course of the next week the normal daily course of activities provided a steady stream of distraction from my thoughts about those embryos, though when the kids were finally asleep in bed and I had a quiet moment to myself, my first thoughts were of those tiny seeds of hope planted inside me, and I wondered expectantly whether they were flourishing or withering away. Time passed quickly until I checked in as scheduled a week later at a local lab for a blood test, and again several days later to monitor my human chorionic gonadotropin (hCG) levels. Lauren called me the following day to share the results Dr. Wilcox had received from the lab.

"Your hCG levels registered relatively high and are climbing rapidly. So, Dr. Wilcox says it looks like we're pregnant!" she cried excitedly.

All four of us! I sat down, slightly shaken, relieved and hopeful all at the same time. It marked the first time that I had really admitted to myself how deeply I had counted on making the first transfer attempt a successful one.

"Really? Wow, that's great! I'm so glad it worked!" I cried back. And smiling to myself, I mused about how oddly new and unique it was to have someone else tell me over the phone that I was pregnant. While it might have been my body, it would not be my pregnancy alone this time around; how intimately thrilling it had been already to share the joy of the news with the new mother-to-be.

I called Robert immediately after I hung up with Lauren to share the news, and I heard the relief in his voice as well, both of us cheered to be able to continue moving forward toward our goal, avoiding the depressing fate of a return all the way back to ground zero. I spoke by phone with Henry later that night to marvel at our incredible luck.

"Congratulations!" I said excitedly.

"Same to you, Pam," Henry responded evenly, and I sensed his see-saw of emotions vacillating between exhilaration and prudent concern. He had, after all, thoroughly researched every angle, every outcome, and every possible point of failure after facing the possibility of losing his wife to cancer. I did not blame him for his reluctance to celebrate; in fact, I welcomed his practical and restrained approach. We had leapt over another hurdle, maybe the biggest one, but there still remained a long road ahead of us littered with anxiety surrounding the unknown. He had the right, the privilege, to worry about the well-being of those embryos. And his concern relieved some of the burden of worrying from my shoulders.

We shared our preliminary success with our parents and a few close friends. (Unfortunately, we unwittingly surrounded Lauren that weekend at a birthday party at our house with those same friends who knew I might be carrying her child; trapping her in a rather awkward moment of unwanted attention.) Of course we told the children the news too, and when they learned the embryo transfer had succeeded, that it indeed appeared that a baby had started growing inside me, they cheered excitedly. We cautioned them that we had to wait a couple more weeks before the doctor could confirm the pregnancy when he searched for a heartbeat, and they voiced their wishes for it to be true, echoing the sentiments of all of us.

"Mommy, I hope there's really a baby in there," Kellie whispered to me earnestly. Though she did not ask me a lot of questions or talk with anyone else about what grew inside my belly, she was my "thinker" and I observed her listening carefully to any discussion Robert and I had about those embryos, considering deeply the meaning and the conse-quences of a successful transfer.

For two weeks we hoped and wondered about our seeming victory with restrained excitement, until September 27th when Robert and I traveled back to Los Angeles, finally meeting Henry and Lauren at the fertility clinic for an ultrasound to search for a heartbeat that would confirm a pregnancy.

As Dr. Wilcox gelled up the ultrasound paddle and slid the smooth metal back and forth across my abdomen, we collectively held our breath as we strained to listen for a discernable sound. The background whoosh of static was soon interrupted by a rapid pounding pulse.

"There it is!" Dr. Wilcox cried.

"Oh, my goodness!" Lauren exclaimed.

She and Henry froze in awe when they heard the quickening of that fetal heart, sending them irrefutable evidence with every beat that the miracle had worked. They were going to have a baby. Though I had heard that same sound three times previously, sharing that moment with another couple brought tears to my eyes, while I witnessed the sense of overwhelming reality settling into their eyes, hearts, and souls. And I, for one, sighed with relief when we heard just one heartbeat that day.

I watched Henry and Lauren, though deeply thrilled, hesitate to embrace their excitement openly, as they recognized there remained a long road ahead before they could hold a healthy bundle of baby in their arms. But I felt confident based on past history that once my body had accepted their embryo, I was well-equipped to nurture and protect it for the long run, and the odds appeared stacked in our favor for me to deliver a baby to Henry and Lauren in May.

Though I had imagined the realization of this moment and believed in the possibility of it all, the indisputable evidence that somehow everything had worked threw me for a loop, albeit a wonderfully exhilarating one. We're really going to have a baby, I thought, the four of us. Now what? I felt some of the burden on my shoulders relieved, but now I thought things might get a little complicated, as I wondered how exactly this would work with the four of us entangled around a joint pregnancy.

But, more importantly, I thought, regardless of the complications and despite the challenges of infertility, Henry would become a dad, and Lauren would become a mom just in time for Mother's Day. I smiled all the way home in the car that afternoon, failing to notice the traffic streaming by or even the curve of the road, lost in thoughts of the baby growing inside me: their baby. Wow. I had managed to come through for them after all.

THE FIRST TRIMESTER

Sharing The Pregnancy

A FEW DAYS LATER BACK AT HOME, Duncan's kindergarten teacher asked the children to create a family drawing in class. When Duncan extracted the slightly crumpled drawing assignment from the bottom of his backpack that evening, we sat down on the couch together to admire it, and I asked him to explain the mysterious identity of each of the colorful stick figures standing at attention on the paper.

He proudly identified himself and then each of his sisters, all drawn according to relative size. He pointed out Daddy, the tall one smiling lopsidedly, and me, sporting round eyes and a few strands of haphazard yellow hair, looking like a frightened scarecrow. Dominating my portrait, however, appeared thick black crayon marks boldly drawn across my middle. Curious, I inquired of Duncan as to the nature of those strange markings.

"Oh. That's my baby cousin, Mommy!" he answered.

"Is that what you told Ms. Warren?" I asked hesitantly.

"Yep!" he proudly confirmed.

Oh no. *Lucy you got some splainin' to do!*

While our children had quickly and enthusiastically embraced their cousin-to-be, we had not yet enlightened their teachers with the details of my surrogate pregnancy, and I worried that Duncan's explanation of his drawing had seriously startled Ms. Warren, a sweet, energetic young woman in her second year of teaching kindergarten. Perhaps, wise to the frequent creative interpretations of five year olds, she had written off Duncan's comments to wishful thinking or a juvenile misunderstanding. Or perhaps Lori Warren had ascertained that Duncan had seemed to be quite clear on the fact that his mother carried his cousin in her belly, and she had chosen to ignore the possible frightening implications. Our *need to know basis* for public disclosure on the surrogacy had clearly come into effect in this case, and I met with Lori the following day after school to inform her about the surrogacy and shed light on the possible cousin confusion.

"Lori, I know Duncan talked to you about my pregnancy, and I just wanted you to know that I am actually carrying his cousin, but as a surrogate for my cousin's wife who had cancer," I explained.

"Oh, wow, o.k.," she said, nodding her head uncertainly.

Though able to clarify the truth on that occasion, I am quite sure that as soon as I walked out of her classroom that afternoon my explanation had only served to generate many more unanswered questions, appearing like a barrage of sequential on-line pop-up windows.

A select few close friends and family members had been providing their love and support for our decision to pursue surrogacy since long before the embryo transfer, but we had never chosen to make a formal announcement to our family or sought to systematically disclose the surrogacy to all of our friends like a to-do list. Instead we spoke personally, one on one, with most each and every one when the appropriate opportunity arose, sharing the journey like a treasured gift, unwrapped carefully and given in confidence. We did not ask for their approval, but we had hoped to receive their support. Often we were bombarded with their curiosity and admiration, usually following an initial awkward, surprised silence.

As we progressed through the transfer and into a successful pregnancy, quickly the number of people aware of the surrogacy began to grow exponentially, particularly when I started enlisting help with carpools and play dates as the combined effects of the continuing hormone regimen and my body's own pregnancy hormones kicked in to wallop me with a serious and unrelenting bout of nausea.

Though I had been "lucky" enough to experience *morning sickness* with all three of my previous pregnancies, I found myself playing in a whole new ballgame with the surrogate pregnancy. I felt like a limp strand of spaghetti, weak and useless. Throwing up became a daily ritual, the nausea crippling my ability to accomplish anything but the most necessary, simple tasks, and an excursion to the grocery store or the post office became a dreaded foggy ordeal, though my daily trips to drop off and pick up the kids at least served to distract me from the consuming sickness in the pit of my belly. I tried and failed with every natural anti-nausea remedy recommended to me, finally resigning myself to just waiting it out, taking some comfort in knowing that the required hormones for a healthy pregnancy apparently raged abundantly inside my aching body. I learned to survive on the bland palette of toast, mashed potatoes, and the occasional cottage cheese, usually washed down with a glass of bubbly ginger ale in a vain attempt to settle the contents of my queasy stomach.

While I lay there listlessly on the couch like a sick dog day after day, Duncan often chose to seek out a more stimulating environment on afternoon play dates with his new kindergarten friends. He unwittingly hastened the widening of the circle of the surrogacy-informed one afternoon when he responded to an inquiry about my pregnancy from the mother of his new friend, Logan.

"So are you excited about having a baby brother or sister?" Logan's mother, Marie, innocently asked Duncan.

"Well, we're not going to keep it because it's my cousin," Duncan replied matter-of-factly, no doubt providing her with a different response then she bargained for.

"Oh!" she mustered in confused response. Marie, given her sensitivity to discretion and privacy, never questioned me on Duncan's statement until months later, when I shared with her the nature of the surrogacy. Today we are good friends who enjoy sharing an array of family secrets over a glass of red wine or a special-recipe margarita, and we joke occasionally about Duncan's conversation-stopping comment and her subsequent hesitancy to expose her son to our family's apparent inbreeding dynamics. I can't say I blame her.

Henry and Lauren shared the surrogacy with their close friends and family, but still retained the ability to control the distribution of that private information at their discretion, as they remained physically removed from the surrogacy's day to day presence.

I know Lauren would have welcomed the opportunity to be the one enduring morning sickness and fielding the pregnancy questions, but absent that possibility, I continued to speak several times a week with both of them to let them in on any updates, grateful for their encouragement and appreciation. As well as providing them with a running commentary on my physical state, I enjoyed rehashing some of my choice encounters apprising random people of the surrogacy. Lauren and I often shared a "*Whatever!*" and a chuckle over some of the more colorful reactions, bonding more closely as we helped each other overcome the incidental discomfort associated with the attention spotlighting our unique, sometimes awkward situation.

Though the majority of our friends, acquaintances and strangers responded admiringly and supportively to my surrogacy, there were an occasional few who simply remained silent, presuming to judge my decision to be a surrogate as immoral or unnatural or preferring to keep their distance for other reasons of discomfort associated with the idea of carrying another person's baby. I never suffered any direct personal attacks, and though I think I would have been disappointed if someone close to me had voiced their discontent, my certainty about the virtue of my choice would have prevented me from ever rethinking the decision to engage in surrogacy.

At the beginning of October I traveled on another train headed for Los Angeles to meet Henry and Lauren for a final visit to the fertility clinic. Though thankful to avoid driving for two hours in L.A traffic, I felt particularly sick and exhausted that morning as I stepped into the train compartment in Solana Beach, and I dreaded riding out the motion of the rails. I slumped into the first empty seat I found, near the bathroom door in case I should feel the sudden urge to use the facilities, and I barely made it the fifteen minutes to Oceanside before I stumbled into the lavatory and kneeled on the rough metal floor with my head hanging over the sterile metal toilet bowl. I endured the rest of the trip slouched in my seat like a rag doll, willing myself not to vomit again as the swaying motion of the rail car added insult to injury.

I limped off the train in downtown Los Angeles like the invalid I had become, shuffling down the ramp and through the echoing tunnel, out to the blindingly sunny station entrance where Lauren waited for me. Blessedly relieved to escape that train ride from hell, I let my eyes close and rested my aching head back against the seat of her car. Lauren eyed my sympathetically. I knew that she and Henry felt badly about the unpleasant intrusion of the surrogacy-related nausea I had been enduring. I am sure had hoped that carrying their child would be as easy, enjoyable, and unobtrusive as possible for me, and I could see them cringe guiltily at times when the surrogacy made me physically uncomfortable.

As I rested there in the front seat of Lauren's car, I asked myself if

I would have offered to be a surrogate had I known how sick I would feel those first few months. Honestly, was it worth it? I loathed surrendering to the grip of nausea's internal waves of sour sickness, and I would have done almost anything to avoid them. But after a moment's pause considering the alternatives, I answered myself in the affirmative quickly and decisively because, despite my physical unease, my heart remained focused on the end goal. My cousin longed for a child, and my offer to him had been a promise sacred as a wedding vow, *in sickness and in health*; no amount of discomfort had diminished my desire to fulfill his wish. I must admit, though, the nausea had seriously compromised the joy of pregnancy over the last several weeks.

The train trip to Los Angeles proved to be worthwhile, however, when Dr. Wilcox rewarded us that day with Henry and Lauren's first baby ultrasound pictures. They now held in their hands visible evidence of the reality of the pregnancy, another weapon for wiping away any lingering doubts about the feasibility of the surrogacy. I took infinite pride and joy in observing them both smiling serenely as they gazed lovingly at their baby in-utero, a miracle they had created together with a little help from a team of medical professionals and my welcoming uterus.

"Congratulations, my job is done," Dr. Wilcox pronounced proudly. "I am releasing your care into the hands of your obstetrician."

I returned home to tape the black and white uterine snapshots to our refrigerator door later that afternoon, pausing to trace gratifyingly the outlines of the life I had helped will into existence, the result of our audacity to hope, to join together and persevere beyond cancer, beyond infertility. I admired the discernable fetal features until long after the edges of the paper had started to curl and the image had faded to a washy gray, and in his excitement, Henry scanned those images immediately after returning to the office that afternoon proudly e-mailing them out to friends and family all over the country.

I scheduled my first appointment with my obstetrician, Dr. Gerber for a couple of weeks later, and rallied in the interim, despite feeling like a train wreck, so that I could attend an annual trip with my college buddies from Stanford. Girls Weekend had become a cherished ritual, initiated several years back, and I had not missed out on one yet. I refused to forgo it this year, desperately looking forward to the relaxing couple of days with my girlfriends as a distraction from the pregnancy. The ten of us would be meeting in the Napa Valley for a weekend of wine tasting, spa treatments, and fine dining.

Unfortunately, none of those pampering pleasures sounded particularly appealing to me given my physical state, but it hardly mattered because the beauty of the weekend, as always, would be the down time to indulge in both meaningful and meaningless chatter with old friends. Every year the days together served as a spiritual retreat where our minds were stimulated, our spirits restored and our enthusiasm rejuvenated, where new ideas took root, old times were revisited, and friends reached out to each other to form a human safety net, catching whomever might be falling, bouncing around whomever needed shaking up, and sending back up to soar those who needed the encouragement to fly. I practically ached for their support this year.

I flew up to the Bay Area on a Thursday afternoon, my surrogacy tools safely packed like a survival kit in the carry-on at my side, though the hormones and syringes which replaced the more typical survival accoutrements of flashlight, batteries, and water would not have been much help in the event of an *emergency water landing*. My Dad picked me up at the airport and took me to take me to my parents' house, where I was spending the night before driving up to Napa the next morning. I enjoyed dinner that evening alone with my Mom and Dad, the relative quiet a departure from the cacophonous family chatter at home and a reminder of the thousands of quiet late night dinners I had partaken in that same kitchen growing up: Mom serving me dinner alone after a daily four-hour gymnastics practice, my three siblings already peacefully slumbering in bed after a much earlier dinner.

After dinner Mom agreed willingly to take Robert's place in delivering my hormone injection, and I meticulously reviewed with her the shot procedure while I prepared the syringe.

"O.k., Mom, go," I prompted.

I leaned on the bathroom counter as Mom eyed her target and then plunged the needle in mercilessly, slamming the syringe hard into my buttocks, like she was trying to pierce elephant hide. *Oh. My. God.* Gritting my teeth through the pain, I suggested, urgently, "O.k., Mom, it's in! You're done! You can take the syringe out now, GENTLY."

"Are you sure," she asked.

"Yes! And I swear I am never going to let you get near me again with a needle in your hand!" I barked at her.

While I had appreciated growing up that my mother never coddled us, and, in fact, I now treated my own children's daily medical emergencies with the same lack of drama, matter-of-factly dispensing a band-aid and quick pat on the head at the sight of blood, I wished for a moment that she had been a little less pragmatic and a little more intimidated by that needle.

In her defense, Mom apologized profusely after the shot, and though I chastised her mercilessly, I eventually thanked her for performing as a willing assistant. Being the sister of Henry's mother, my Mom treasured her connection to her nephew, and having sympathized compassionately when apprised of Lauren's struggle with cancer and her consequent infertility, she and my Dad had supported wholeheartedly my decision to offer my help in becoming a surrogate for Henry and Lauren. In our conversation later that night regarding the practical realities of my surrogate pregnancy, I could see that my commitment to giving their nephew the chance of a family moved them intimately.

The next day I drove lazily up to Napa on a beautiful fall morning (a forgiving drivers seat thankfully cushioning my sore butt), in delighted anticipation of meeting the girls at a *villa* we had rented for the weekend.

Greeting each other amidst a reunion of hugs and squeals of delight in the driveway, we ventured inside and eyed amusingly our accommodations. The house had photographed well from the exterior for the Internet, but its location and bizarre mix of interior décor inspired more of a comparison to the Winchester Mystery House than one with that month's featured Italian villa in the Conde Nast Traveler magazine. No matter, or "pee-shaw", as Sherri, one of the girls, often said: it would prove easy enough to overlook the oddities and ignore the inconvenience while we reveled in the time together. We could make ourselves comfortable chatting late into the night curled up on saggy couches or mixed up in a pile of old pillows on a worn shag carpet. Just leave us together with some blankets and a wine opener.

We enjoyed a relaxing day with leisurely shopping as the background for a nonstop stream of animated conversation, punctuated by exclamations of surprise, joy, and sympathy, the stories spilling over uninterrupted into a tasting venture at a local winery, when sampling the wine forced everyone to at last take a breath between stories. (Well, that is except for me. Even a whiff of the wine my friends sipped sent me reeling to the porch balcony.)

We returned to the villa together that evening for a gourmet dinner prepared by a local chef, a blessed indulgent break for each of us from the monotony of throwing together family meals. What a relief to be on vacation! We sat around the dinner table that night talking until the wee hours of the morning: sharing funny stories, confessing secrets from our Stanford days, and comparing the real or exaggerated inadequacies of our husbands. Finally, unable to keep my eyes open any longer, I excused myself to bed, recruiting a reluctant Shelli, who is like a sister to me, to perform the injection honors for me that night.

I demonstrated the procedure and then handed over the filled syringe, offering her encouragement as she worked up the nerve to plunge it in. Finally, after a few dry runs, she quickly poked in the needle timidly while peering through half-shut eyelids. When she opened her eyes, she found to her horror that she had struck a vein, causing blood to spurt in a sustained arc onto the bathroom floor, a surreal red fountain spouting from my butt cheek. Glimpsing my backside in the mirror, I imagined myself posing statuesquely among the formal hedges in the garden of a nobleman with a macabre sense of humor. (Except my behind failed to resemble the beautiful chiseled hardness of the lustrous sculpted marble creations of Luca della Robia and the other Italian masters we had studied together at Stanford's campus in Florence.)

"Ahhhhh! You're bleeding!" Shelli screamed, mortified.

After calmly assuring her that I felt no pain, I coaxed her into completing the shot, instructing her to grab hold of the flopping syringe and push it in fully to release the hormones before removing the needle. To stem the blood flow, she frantically threw open cabinets and grabbed toilet paper, Kleenex and paper towels as fast as she could. As I applied pressure to the wound with the haphazard wad of sanitary materials, Shelli mopped up the blood-spattered floor with wet rags, apologizing repeatedly.

"Please don't ever ask me to do that again!" she begged.

We laughed about it together half-heartedly, and, wide-eyed, she retreated from the bathroom like a sheepish dog, relieved that the ordeal had ended. Though the errant shot had proved to be only a minor mishap, I looked forward to returning home, where I could rely on my husband to administer my daily jabs without incident.

During our many opportunities for group and private conversation that weekend, my friends voiced their concerns about the surrogacy while they questioned me face to face, determined to probe my emotional health in the midst of a trying first trimester carrying another mother's child.

"Does it feel strange to carry someone else's baby? Does it feel like it's yours? Are you worried about becoming attached to it or about how you will feel watching the baby grow up?" my friends asked in succession.

Though my belly had not yet begun to expand enough to *show*, and it would be weeks before I could feel the baby inside of me, the questions posed reflected my own curiosity about the beginnings of the surrogacy. While I had not found it to this point strange or unnatural to carry someone else's baby, I realized I related differently to this pregnancy from my previous ones. Although attached to this baby both physically and emotionally, I recognized that our attachment failed to imitate the mother-child bond I had experienced in-utero with my own three children.

"Knowing this baby is not mine, my thoughts are just more focused on safeguarding the life inside of me rather than nurturing a connection for the future," I explained. Though the girls accepted my explanation, I think at least a few of them failed to grasp the ability to emotionally distinguish between different kinds of pregnancies.

"Is Robert okay with it? My husband says he doesn't think he would have let me do that," another friend commented.

This question caught me a little off-guard, because although I had asked Robert for his approval and support with the surrogacy, I had never seriously considered that he would be so uncomfortable with it that he might withhold his permission for me to follow my desire to pursue a surrogate relationship with my cousin. And while the surrogacy would obviously be much more fulfilling with Robert's unconditional support, I could not imagine letting his hesitation or discomfort deprive me of the opportunity to engage in a quest that held so much meaning for me, at least not without a fight. Well, therein lay the problem, though. If I had been forced to fight Robert for the surrogacy, then perhaps I would have had to reconsider, because jeopardizing the harmony of my marriage to help my cousin create his own family inevitably would have been self-destructive.

"Thankfully, Robert is very supportive of the surrogacy, and seems just as excited about it as I am," I answered appreciatively.

"Do you feel like Henry and Lauren really appreciate what you are going through for them?" someone else asked. Tough question.

While I knew they greatly appreciated my offer and recognized the sacrifices I had made to be their surrogate, I considered it impossible for them to really understand what it meant for me to carry their pregnancy without having personally experienced a pregnancy themselves. Just like a husband might sympathize but cannot *empathize* with his wife's pregnancy, it would not be possible for an intended couple either; in fact they are even further removed since they are not there on day-by-day basis experiencing even second-hand the implications of carrying a child around inside twenty-four hours a day for nine months. Admittedly, I wished it were possible for them to truly know what that meant.

"Henry and Lauren let me know on a regular basis with their words and actions how much they appreciate me and my efforts, though," I assured my friends.

And that deep appreciation, without which I would have resented the shots, the time required, the debilitating nausea and the other difficult moments of the pregnancy, was, in fact, what proved to make our surrogacy so worthwhile and meaningful.

"Are you worried about the birth and giving up the baby?" a friend inquired.

Quite honestly I had not given much thought yet to the actual birth since the pregnancy still remained relatively new and we had several long months before we would reach that chapter of the surrogacy. Besides, I had given birth three times previously. And though I wondered if the transition might present some unique challenges, given that I expected to form some kind of attachment to Henry and Lauren's child, truthfully no conflicting emotions about giving up a baby were rattling around uncomfortably inside my head.

"I will be giving *back* a baby. The baby has never belonged to me," I explained.

In addition to the scientific point of fact that I could not claim to be the biological mother of the child inside me, in my mind the mother was not the one who carried the child; my body was simply acting as a vessel for the baby's journey into life. The mother was the one who willfully set out to welcome a new life into the world, who nurtured the child with unconditional love, responded to every tear, scrape and disappointment and rejoiced in every success and cause for celebration. That intent and privilege belonged to Lauren and Henry, not to me.

Though my answers to their questions sincerely expressed my deepest feelings about the surrogacy, I felt like I had failed to adequately communicate the emotional context of the pregnancy or cogently illuminate the differences from a traditional pregnancy for some of my closest friends. Perhaps, rather than my lack of effective communication, it was the intimately personal nature of surrogacy that for others, without their own experience, had made comprehensive understanding impossible. Perhaps it was somewhat like an astronaut trying to explain how it felt to fly up to the moon and look back at Earth from a whole new perspective.

Despite their inability to grasp a comprehensive understanding of the surrogacy, my friends still expressed with unconditional love their relief to find me stable and optimistic, swarming me with greatly appreciated warm hugs, heartfelt words of admiration for my courage and compassion, and sincere encouragement for a successful journey.

Physically, that weekend proved to be almost more than I could handle, but the mental boost and emotional restoration I had enjoyed from an outing with dear friends far outweighed the inconveniences. I had not admitted to myself how much I had needed that weekend, a chance to let go for a few days the need to be strong, instead allowing myself to depend on my friends for nourishment and strength, regrouping and reconfirming for myself my ability to complete my long voyage. In short, that weekend gave me a break from the pressure and responsibility of delivering a miracle. Surrogacy truly demands a strong support network of family and friends to carry you through, and boy am I lucky to count them in spades.

Another, more formal support group of women reached out to me with the insider's perspective on the surrogacy later that month: a group of surrogates the psychologist, Karen Chernekoff, met with on a monthly basis in San Diego. Karen invited me to join them at their October meeting the following week at a restaurant in Carlsbad, and with Robert's supportive encouragement (no doubt because he hoped it would help preserve my sanity), I decided with some curiosity to attend.

In the back corner of a nondescript chain restaurant, I listened that night to a group of compassionate surrogates sharing their stories, concerns, hopes and frustrations from their quests to help deliver children to expectant intended parents.

These were strong, determined women, confident and comfortable in their decision to carry someone else's child. A surrogacy agency had screened each of the six women and matched them with a couple, and each had experienced inevitable delays that had crippled their attempts to become surrogates, frustrations which I had never faced: difficulties finding an optimal match with a couple, communication snafus with couples living across the country and the world, and obstacles encountered in timing cycles correctly and conveniently for receiving a fresh embryo transfer. Other difficulties they encountered, including recent miscarriages and commonplace failed transfer attempts, I had escaped by pure luck.

I found myself embarrassed, in fact, on some level, to share my story when Karen asked me to relay the positive news of my pregnancy to triumph the heavy burden of negative news that night, embarrassed because we had become pregnant relatively easily. My reality: I knew and loved my intended couple, we lived close enough to visit often and talked easily, and I had conceived a successful and viable pregnancy on the first attempt. I felt like I had cheated. I did not really deserve to be there, I thought; I did not really belong.

I sat there anyway, though, listening to the stories of those courageous women that night as they leaned on each other for sympathy and support while they navigated the more traditional path of a surrogate, and I marveled at their choice to endure a mountain of trouble and heartache in the hopes of relieving relative strangers of the burden of infertility and giving them the wonder of a family. I could lay claim to some extent the same kind of altruistic motives as the other women in the room, but, in fact, I knew the baby I carried would bring joy to my extended family, and indirectly by extension, joy in the end to me.

While they expressed hope that they would have periodic communication with the family in the baby's first year, they had no expectations beyond that, focusing instead on their present connection with the couple they were so determined to help. I could expect, though, or hope for at least, the occasional reward of watching the baby inside me grow up at family gatherings and of witnessing first-hand the ongoing joy of my cousin's chance to be a father and Lauren's opportunity to experience the joys of motherhood. Though the surrogate pregnancy would end my direct connection to the baby, I would never have to say a final goodbye.

Yes, it is true that hopeful couples would be compensating these other women with a significant amount of money for acting as surrogates, somewhere in the neighborhood of $15,000 to $20,000 or more, and that compensation was surely a factor in their choices to become surrogates. When you consider, though, that such payment amounts to cents on the hour over the course of a year for which they give up their lifestyle, time and energy to accept the medical risks and 24 hour a day commitment of surrogacy, you realize quickly that the money cannot be the primary motivator. Instead, these women offer themselves up as surrogates for the intended parents in a selfless, extraordinary act of giving, expecting in exchange only boundless appreciation. The bonus of compensation simply gave these women the hard-earned chance to invest in a better future for their own family.

Though I failed to follow the traditional path to becoming a surrogate, there were still ways in which I fit the profile of a typical surrogate mom: strong and stable mentally to withstand the constant challenges of surrogacy, flexible to gracefully accept the complexities of sharing a pregnancy, and willing to make sacrifices of my time and body for a greater purpose. Like many other surrogates, I harbored a desire to accomplish something remarkable with my life, viewing surrogacy as a unique opportunity to make a contribution and achieve a sense of self-actualization. When or how else could I make such a huge, direct, personal impact on someone's life? And, of course, all of us hoped to arrive at the same destination: the delivery of a baby who would be the miracle for which the intended parents hoped so desperately.

Even though my experience matched unevenly with that of the other surrogates in the group, many of the emotional, social, psychological and physical considerations and challenges still remained similar, and my experience resonated with them that night as we voiced our feelings about our surrogacy experiences. In that safe space of mutual understanding, we could share our concerns and complaints without feeling guilty about being selfish. Listening to each other gave us the credence and permission to be frustrated, without the need to act positive or brave when we felt otherwise, because we were afraid someone might take it the wrong way and think we regretted our decisions to be surrogates. Our conversation helped us understand that what we were thinking and feeling was normal, not irrational or damaging or self-serving.

Though these women represented a group of relative strangers with whom I had shared no past or friendship, we all felt the underlying connection and immediate understanding that comes from engaging in a similar experience. And so they accepted my feelings, my motivations, my frustrations without question: no explanations required. I emerged from the restaurant meeting that evening thankful for the strength and boost of confidence I derived from the opportunity to speak with women who had a fundamental understanding of what it meant, what it really felt like, to act as a surrogate. And my success story of a viable pregnancy offered them hope that night that they would eventually be successful in their own quests.

A couple of weeks later I attended with Henry and Lauren the first appointment with my obstetrician in Encinitas, Dr. Gerber, a neighbor and a parent of a child in Duncan's kindergarten class.

Though I had been unsure of exactly how she might respond to the idea of a surrogate pregnancy, I greatly admired Dr. Gerber's care and bedside manner, and I had informed her of our unique situation confident in her ability to manage our surrogacy smoothly. I hoped that with time to prepare herself for the more complex care of a surrogate, she would become comfortable with and excited about the opportunity to facilitate our journey, minimizing the awkwardness of our shared experience with the intended parents and multiple extended families over the course of the pregnancy and delivery.

On our first appointment that day at the clinic, Lauren and Henry sat in the waiting room while Dr. Gerber's nurse assistant accompanied me into the examining room to question me confidentially on my obstetrical history. She checked boxes and took notes on my previous pregnancies and deliveries, rattling off questions with administrative efficiency:

"How many previous pregnancies?" she asked

"Three," I answered.

"How many live births," she asked.

"Three," I answered.

"Dates of birth? Birth weights? Sex?" she asked in succession.

And I provided her with answers one after the other, as she ran down her list diligently, until her querying changed direction.

"Is your husband the father of this pregnancy?" she asked me routinely.

"No. Actually, my cousin is the father of the baby," I answered.

Having disrupted the impassive flow of her questioning, I watched her look up from her clipboard, pen frozen in mid-air, eyebrows raised in a confused, hesitant expression, not sure if she should be mortified or fascinated. I refrained from helping her out by filling in the blanks and explaining the surrogacy to her, entertained by her frantic attempt to sort through that bit of information. Instead I challenged her with the next bit of news and waited for the reaction.

"And I am not the mother of the baby," I continued, hesitating momentarily when she screwed up her face in puzzlement, "but a surrogate for my cousin's wife," I finally explained further.

I chose not to provide her with any further information to accommodate her certain questions, not yet ready or willing to share that story, and so she proceeded to scribble several words in the margins of my chart, covering up her surprise with suddenly intense note taking. Obviously, Dr. Gerber had not apprised her yet of the situation, and amused to observe her shaken composure, I smiled to myself as she stood there awkwardly trying to recover from the shock as she completed her interview.

Lauren and Henry joined me a few moments later in a room down the hall, as we waited for Dr. Gerber to come examine my belly.

"Hi, everybody; nice to see you, Pam," she said as she walked in the room. "I'm Dr. Gerber," she introduced herself to Henry and Lauren.

Welcoming all of us warmly, she appeared shy and uncertain initially as she shared her perspective on pregnancy and delivery, but after her initial hesitation about to whom she should direct the discussion, she became comfortable speaking openly with all three of us, directing pertinent information about the baby and the pregnancy to Henry and Lauren as the parents and to me as the patient.

Because Dr. Gerber would be guiding all of us through the anxious moments of pregnancy and delivery over the next several months to bring this baby safely into the world, I felt relieved to see that Henry and Lauren appeared at ease with her. Moved by our trust in choosing her, and truly touched and humbled, I believe, by the journey I had embarked upon with my cousin, Dr. Gerber felt compelled in that introductory visit to voice her unquestionable support for the surrogacy. And observing her during the course of that visit, I knew in my gut we had picked the right doctor; a kind, respectful soul to join us on our journey.

As we stepped out the inner door of the office with the examination and introductions completed, I overheard the flurried beginnings of hushed inquiry from the nurse and other staff. "Did you hear that she is carrying her cousin's baby?" someone whispered incredulously from down the hall.

Gestational surrogacy, first performed successfully in 1985, is becoming more common as the success rates of assisted reproductive technology continue to climb, allowing thousands of couples to fulfill their dreams of a child, but is still rare and unexpected even in a busy OB's office where they care for hundreds of pregnancies every year. Clearly we would be a novelty in this office.

After our appointment that morning Lauren and Henry dropped me off at the house with an assortment of accessories that Lauren had hunted down for the kids' Halloween costumes. The hormones were still kicking my butt, literally and figuratively and I lacked my usual stamina; for two more weeks I would be required to continue the hormone regimen of shots, patches and lozenges. Lauren had generously offered to save me from shuffling down shop aisles, afraid of *losing my lunch* while searching in vain for costume accoutrements.

She elevated shopping to an art form with the uncanny ability to find that perfect item, and Kellie, in particular, appeared thrilled with the mouse ears and purple plastic purse for her "Lily" costume, parading around the house that entire afternoon like author Kevin Henkes' storybook mouse princess. It felt like a natural exchange of compassionate assistance: they took care of me and my kids when I did not feel up to it, and I took care of their baby growing inside me.

Though I encountered moments during this first trimester when I fleetingly second-guessed my decision to become a surrogate as I suffered through a debilitating pregnancy while caring for my three young children, wishing aloud sometimes for the damned nausea to let me go, Henry and Lauren demonstrated a care, involvement and understanding from day one of the surrogacy that rendered those moments inconsequential and impermanent, leaving no trace of bitterness. Instead of resenting my compromised ability to be a fully functional Mom, I came to appreciate Lauren's offers of help, and while of course she could not replace me, the kids learned from her too, and most importantly learned from both of us about the joy and self-fulfillment that comes from caring for others.

And, in addition to sensitive and supportive intended parents, I knew I could rely on Robert to be a committed and enthusiastic partner in the surrogacy. In the midst of his demanding work schedule, Robert picked up the significant slack I left in the wake of my immobility, assuming the primary caretaker role and cooking most of the dinners that fall, completing numerous loads of laundry, hammering out the shopping and heading up the daily bedtime ritual. I felt deeply grateful to have him at my side, though I knew he was often exhausted and desperate for me to be fully functional again. Surrogacy proved to be a group effort. Even the kids played a vital role, summoning patience, compassion and understanding at a young age when they found they could not depend on Mom to respond immediately to their needs, often selflessly offering a foot rub or a hug or a can of 7-up when I needed it most.

"It's okay, Mommy," Lise often said, stroking my cheek and patting my head, a comforting gesture from a sympathetic three year-old.

While I dreaded lying on the couch day after day, willing my body not to give in to the nausea, I knew that eventually it had to end and I held on to the hope that soon I might be able to enjoy the surrogacy more comfortably. In the middle of November, a couple of weeks removed from completing the hormone shot regimen (yes!), with the pregnancy dependent solely on my body for producing and delivering the necessary hormones, the nausea finally began to loosen its grip. In addition to family and friendship, I would count my recovering appetite as something to be thankful for at Thanksgiving that year. And Robert could celebrate with weary thankfulness the end to his services as an in-home nurse.

The week before Thanksgiving Lauren drove down from Los Angeles with her Mom, Joyce, to attend another appointment with our obstetrician. I had hoped that by meeting Dr. Gerber first-hand and having the opportunity to ask her any pressing questions, Joyce would come to feel like she was more a part of the pregnancy, easing some of the apprehension she must have felt about the surrogacy.

I knew that Lauren's battle with cancer had frightened Joyce, and though she was relieved that Lauren had survived the disease, she still mourned the devastating loss of her daughter's ability to carry her own babies. I hoped, though that in time she would overcome her disappointment and come to embrace our surrogacy. Though a woman is designed to give birth, pregnancy itself is a singular nine-month experience which does not define motherhood; instead, in fact, I believe it is the commitment to embracing that role every moment after the end of the nine months that defines a mother and matters most. I hoped Lauren's Mom would come to focus instead on that opportunity for her daughter.

For the second visit, Dr. Gerber's assistant and the rest of the office staff appeared to be more comfortable with serving the doctor's first surrogacy, and they treated us with respectful admiration and curiosity, welcoming Joyce, the intended grandmother, like a celebrity into the examining room that day.

"The pregnancy is progressing beautifully, and though Pam has barely gained any weight due to the nausea, there is no need to be concerned for the baby," Dr. Gerber confirmed for us.

The three of us smiled thankfully, and I sensed Joyce's perspective shifting subtly. Her presence at that OB appointment seemed to be an important step in her reconciliation with Lauren's cancer, and the first seeds of excitement about a new baby appeared to germinate cautiously within her.

After our appointment, Lauren and Joyce drove me to Solana Beach for lunch at an outdoor café just down the street from the dreaded train. Having overcome the tiresome toilet bowl reflex, I finally worked up enough energy and appetite to eat out for the first time in what seemed like forever. Though it was simply a warm loaf of French bread and a green salad, that meal picked me up like a breath of fresh air. Lauren's mother, a generous, funny lady, entertained us all through lunch with outrageous personal stories told with the panache of a gifted storyteller, and I thoroughly enjoyed that hour of what felt like the first taste of freedom in months, freedom from discomfort and freedom to engage the outside world.

After lunch we strolled across the street to a maternity store, where Lauren insisted on buying me some new clothes, as our first trimester was coming to a close and my belly was beginning to stretch uncomfortably against the waistline of my pants. I had not yet dared to pull out the old bag of pregnancy clothes in my closet, clothes I had long ago become supremely sick and tired of wearing week after week for an endless 27 months altogether, the kind of clothes that inevitably never quite fit or flattered. Thankfully, the fashion industry had finally taken notice of the pregnant woman's predicament, and in the last couple of years had designed and produced fashionable maternity clothing in natural fabrics; no longer were we forced to hide behind unflattering extra yards of synthetic material loosely covering an expanding waistline. I delighted in trying on maternity wear that could actually be considered hip and still fit comfortably and soothingly the new curves of my growing body.

Because my belly would be inflating like a balloon over the course of the pregnancy, I tried the clothes on with one of those strap-on pillows they thoughtfully stock in maternity dressing rooms so mothers-to-be can see how the fit and look will be when they are closer to term.

"Lauren, come on into the dressing room," I invited. "Here, try on one of these pillows with me," I encouraged.

Handing her a pillow, I gave her permission to experience one of the inevitable practicalities of pregnancy, the fitting of a new wardrobe against your own awkward shape that hardly resembles the one with which you are comfortable and familiar. We giggled at ourselves in the dressing room mirror, standing side by side with pillows strapped to our bellies like misplaced life preservers. I enjoyed that silly moment we shared in the pregnancy together. It allowed Lauren a chance to glimpse at least the unique sensation of carrying a baby around your belly, although unfortunately it lacked the true sense of what it is like to hold a life within your womb. I wish I could have given her that too.

Lauren quickly shed the maternity pillow and clothes, uncomfortable pretending for longer than a few minutes to be someone the cancer had rendered a devastating impossibility, and I saw in her mirrored reflection how difficult and awkward this must have been for her to let someone else carry her child, to experience what should have been her right and privilege. I had been focusing on the opportunity and excitement of our journey, forgetting that Lauren, though grateful beyond words, was wishing she had never had to embark upon it. And I recognized then her remarkable bravery in fighting her way through cancer and subsequent infertility, and in giving up control over the future to leave it in my hands, my body. Her courage humbled me.

Lauren bought me some beautiful clothes that afternoon before we stepped out of the shop to pick up the kids at school, and we all arrived back at the house in time for Joyce and Lauren to entertain the kids for a brief time before they had to leave to drive back to Los Angeles in time to avoid rush hour. They thoughtfully left us a home-made lasagna baking in the oven for dinner, so Robert and I could relax without having to summon up the energy required to prepare a warm meal. It was simple act of kindness that felt like a gift from the heavens for an exhausted surrogate and her worn out husband. Joyce and Lauren's attentive care and companionship undeniably reached out and lifted up my spirits that day, and I hoped our continued progress buoyed theirs too.

The following week, three months into the pregnancy, our whole family traveled up to Palos Verdes in *the big blue bus*, our affectionately nicknamed SUV, to celebrate Thanksgiving with Henry, Lauren and Lauren's extended family at her parents' house. Honored to be invited by Lauren's parents, to be included in their family holiday, we arrived into Joyce and Jerry's beautiful home with a warm welcome, the long dining room table set for a festive family gathering, and savory smells of roasted turkey swirling out from under the kitchen doors.

"Come on in and meet everybody," Lauren invited.

We were introduced to cousins, aunts and uncles as we made our way into the house, shedding coats and offering holiday greetings. Circling about the living room and chatting during the cocktail hour, I quickly sensed the relatives' discomfort in my presence, as they eyed me cautiously, stealing furtive looks at my belly, echoing the weary way the Indians and Pilgrims had probably regarded each other hundreds of years before at the first Thanksgiving. Though I had not arrived as a member of a foreign culture from across the Atlantic, it became obvious that the foreign nature of the surrogacy had risen up like an ocean between us.

Although we conversed politely on other topics, the evening passed without one question, comment, or word of congratulations from them on the surrogate pregnancy. While their response (or lack of it) caused me no deep disappointment, it did surprise me, and I hoped it did not suggest an unwillingness to accept the surrogacy. Their response, instead, may have simply reflected the discomfort they felt about discussing openly a topic so personal (and perhaps incomprehensible) with someone they had never met before that night. I had hoped, though, to observe them showering Lauren openly with joy and excitement for her granted chance at motherhood; after all she had been through I felt she deserved their unbridled encouragement. Lauren commented in a whispered aside to me later that evening that their failure to mention the surrogacy seemed a bit strange, but she did not appear to be particularly surprised or concerned by their apprehension toward engaging in a conversation about the child I carried in my belly. The only one who failed to eye me curiously that night proved to be Lauren's blissfully unaware 90 year old grandfather, who had not quite grasped the concept of an embryo transfer when Lauren shared the surrogacy with him some days earlier.

While the absence of public acceptance and congratulations from Lauren's relatives failed to ruffle me much, I did hope for understanding and encouragement from my own extended family. My Grandaddy, a grandfather to both Henry and me, had just celebrated his own 90th birthday, though fortunately with his engineer's mind still live as a wire he had understood well enough to give us both his loving encouragement when he received the news of the surrogacy.

Grandaddy, in fact, held a unique and almost incomprehensible perspective on the surrogacy, as his granddaughter was pregnant with his grandson's child. For a man born in 1910, before radio or television ruled the day, when in-vitro fertilization, the internet, and mobile phones represented the stuff of science fiction (though as a previous AT&T Vice President he had probably seen the cell phone coming long before the rest of us), the creation of his great grandchild must have seemed like a wild fantasy.

But fantasy it was not. At the end of a very real first trimester, the nausea had subsided dramatically, and I was able to enjoy a healthy portion of the elaborate Thanksgiving dinner Joyce had prepared that night. Wrapped in Joyce and Jerry's accepting welcome, I found it encouraging to participate in a family meal again, interacting with other people rather than staying holed up on the couch in the family room relegated to hours of torturous boredom with only myself for company. Kellie serenaded us with an improvisational piano concert that night while we ate our way through turkey, sweet potatoes, pumpkin soup, and loads of pie. The holidays had arrived, and (finally) so had my appetite.

THE SECOND TRiMESTER

This Baby Is Not Mine

STEPPING UP ON THE OFFICE SCALE at our monthly OB appointment with Dr. Gerber on December 7th, I watched with curious anticipation as the nurse slid the metal weights across the hatch marks until the bar achieved a level balance: 134 lbs. So far so good, I assured Lauren, who had driven down to Encinitas to join me for my check-up; I had gained a few pounds and now stood six pounds heavier than my pre-transfer weight, the beginning bulge in my belly visible evidence of continued fetal growth and development. I peed in a cup and submitted to the blood pressure cuff, which was routine monthly testing for any progressing pregnancy, then waited in the patient room for Dr. Gerber to examine me.

Lauren, though happy to be there with me and grateful to be included, observed these visits from a strange outside perspective (as part of her, but not exactly), watching me undergo doctor examinations for what should have been her pregnancy. I tried to make her as comfortable and as much a part of our OB appointments as possible, and though there were the inevitable awkward moments during our visits and the surrogacy as a whole, her excitement about the baby thankfully prevented them from turning our journey into a negative adventure. And Dr. Gerber's approach helped keep her focus positive.

"Pam and the baby are doing great and progressing normally," Dr. Gerber assured Lauren confidently, after examining my belly and measuring its height.

Though in some ways the progression of our surrogacy resembled any typical pregnancy, and the examinations themselves proved routine, I know that our pregnancy presented a sometimes awkward situation for Dr. Gerber as well. She herself carried the pregnancy of her third child, due one month before us, and she had delivered hundreds of babies previously, but still this marked her first time managing a surrogacy. After a bit of initial hesitation about the appropriate approach and protocol for our situation, though, Dr. Gerber intuitively handled our arrangement gracefully and compassionately, quickly becoming a steady source of support and strength for all of us. We trusted her implicitly and she treated our journey as a privileged opportunity; we could not have asked for a better partner.

Lauren and I hugged each other in the parking lot after our brief visit to the doctor's office that December morning, and she headed up North back to Los Angeles for work, as I turned South for an appointment with a masseuse for a much anticipated pregnancy massage. Lauren and Henry had thoughtfully purchased a series of six massages for me to ease the aches of pregnancy, and now that the nausea had lessened, I could finally feel comfortable lying on the therapist's table without worrying about falling victim to the sudden urge to revisit my breakfast.

Slipping under the warm sheets on the massage table, I closed my eyes and took a deep breath, relaxing under the soothing touch of the therapist's hands as they relieved the tension in my aching body, blissfully allowing someone else to take care of me for a bit. I treasured the opportunity to simply lie down for a peaceful hour in semi-dark isolation, removed from the urge to frantically wipe down the kitchen or dash to the grocery store before the kids came home from school; a heavenly respite. Allowing my thoughts to wander freely and uninterrupted while she worked her magic on my muscles and joints for sixty minutes, the stress ebbed away like the receding waves at low tide, and I emerged from that peaceful chamber as relaxed and content as a cat stretching after an afternoon nap in the sun.

The gift of massage from Henry and Lauren acknowledged their appreciation for the daily sacrifices I endured to help them realize their dream of a family; the simple comfort of knowing that they sought creative and thoughtful ways to thank me proved more precious even than the direct benefits of the massage itself. The rewards for the nausea, exhaustion, aches and bodily transformation that had accompanied my previous pregnancies had appeared in the daily strengthening of a bond with the baby inside me and the joy of looking forward to bringing a new life into our family; but the rewards as a surrogate proved less straight forward. I could not wait to give my cousin a family, but that would be months away; in the throes of a surrogate pregnancy, a huge and ever-present commitment, I found I depended heavily on the more immediate daily words and acts of appreciation from Henry and Lauren to nurture me throughout the passage, sometimes trying and inconvenient, on the way to our goal.

While I wrapped Christmas presents and wrote holiday cards as celebration of the holidays kicked into high gear, I paused to think back to the beginning of our voyage at Christmas the year before, when I had presented Henry and Lauren with the gift of surrogacy, not knowing then or even daring to imagine that after deliberating, preparing for and pursuing surrogacy for one whole year, we would be well on our way to their dream of a family. With my energy and thoughts focused on the growing baby inside me, I could appreciate more profoundly the wise words of Dr. Seuss, who suggested through the Grinch's belated revelation that perhaps Christmas is not found in packages, boxes, and bags, but that Christmas is something much bigger, that *Christmas...perhaps*

....means a little bit more. Like the Grinch, I felt my heart expanding in new directions as I looked forward to sharing the miracle of this baby-to-be over the holidays in Tahoe with Henry's family.

On Christmas Day my family piled into *the big blue bus,* driving around Lake Tahoe at the foot of the snow-covered Sierras over to my Aunt Pam's house on the Nevada side, weighed down with gifts and food for Christmas dinner. We reveled that night, as always, in the time to renew family connections, and I delighted in observing Henry and Lauren thrill to the attention on the baby-to-be.

"I wonder who the baby will look like," my cousin, Wende, mused as we relaxed together on the couch stuffed, like the cushions we curled up in, from a dinner of meat, potatoes and pie.

"Let's just hope that it has Lauren's temperament and not Henry's," my father joked, reminiscing about my cousin's wild childhood antics as he stoked the fire.

I sat there, smiling and pregnant, with my Aunt eyeing me appreciatively, while Henry and Lauren received a gift from my sister, Marlene, tiny elf booties for the baby inside me. The true Who-ville Christmas spirit touched me that evening, as my heart rejoiced with the chance to witness the family's excitement for Henry and Lauren, though I managed to refrain from reaching out to hold hands and sing *Welcome Christmas, Christmas Day!*

Though barely showing now, I passed up the chance to ski with everyone else that week as a precaution against the risk of a fall on the slopes that could potentially harm the baby growing inside me. I usually ski relatively cautiously but not flawlessly, and I am always given to at least one face full of snow on each trip (much to the kids' amusement). I could only imagine how devastating it would be for all of us if I took an unnecessary chance that ended our quest prematurely, taking away the very dream I had set out to give Henry and Lauren. No matter how far removed the possibility of a mishap, I preferred to play it safe.

Though I had generally maintained a positive outlook on the surrogacy, truthfully every step of the way I had struggled to suppress my anxiety: worrying my uterus would not accept the embryos, fearing the possibility of miscarriage, and now anxious that some unforeseen accident could yank away our dream. By necessity Henry and Lauren had given up control of the pregnancy and entrusted their baby to me, and I judged it my responsibility to them to consider my actions wisely, proceeding even more cautiously than with my own pregnancies. A speedy run down the side of a mountain covered with snow on two planks of fiberglass would not be worth the risks when I had a life inside me to protect.

Instead, relishing the time to relax by myself in the cabin, I escaped the madness of the ski resorts during the holidays and remained at home, reading by the fire with thoughts of the baby wrapping me in a cloak of contentment. Resting under a blanket cuddled up on the couch in a quiet moment alone, I felt the first flutter of fetal movement inside me. Wow! Whoa! In that instant a physical connection with the baby shifted my focus on the surrogate *pregnancy* to the life growing inside me. With a few kicks the baby communicated to me: Knock, knock. Here I am; I am real. Though I remember this first moment of physical connection and engagement with each of my own children, this time around it touched me differently, because the beginnings of life had been so clinical, and so surreal, that I found it remarkable, yet again, that our *experiment* had actually worked. Somebody else's baby tumbled around inside me.

Though I knew it would be several more weeks before the baby kicked forcefully enough, I found myself looking forward eagerly to sharing with Henry and Lauren the opportunity to feel their child move inside of me. There is an element to touch that connects with reality more tangibly than the other senses, and though they had already marveled at hearing the fetal heartbeat and seeing the ultrasound pictures, I eagerly anticipated the moment when they first experienced a real physical connection to their baby. I hoped that witnessing fetal movement, however cloaked beneath the protective layers of my body, would make this baby's existence more real, more present for Henry and Lauren.

Robert, I and the kids celebrated the 2001 New Year back at home in San Diego, and the following week. On January 8th we arrived back at Dr. Gerber's office with Henry and Lauren, searching for more concrete signs of their baby inside me.

"Do you want to know the sex," Dr. Gerber asked, as she fired up the ultrasound.

"Yes, definitely," Henry and Lauren answered in anticipation.

"Okay, let's see who's in there," she said.

Gliding the gelled paddle across my belly, Dr. Gerber examined the monitor for evidence that would reveal the news Henry and Lauren eagerly awaited. They sat closely together beside me while they watched the baby come into view. Who exactly swam around and kicked inside me?

"It's a healthy baby girl!" Dr Gerber pronounced.

I turned to watch Henry and Lauren smile elatedly, as they guarded that cluster of precious few words as a beacon of hope, holding it in a tight embrace and caressing the bit of news like the miracle it truly represented. Though not directly responsible for the gender of the baby inside me, my body had guided the hand of destiny in choosing which embryo to embrace, and I proudly welcomed the delightful news of a little girl.

"Oh, my goodness! We're having a girl!" Lauren exclaimed.

Henry's eyes sparkled with promise. It was at that moment, absorbing the news and imagining their future with a daughter, that I felt their consciousness shift to fully embrace the baby inside of me. The highly anticipated announcement provided them with a concrete vision to prepare for mentally and physically, making more tangible the reality that a new baby would be arriving in their lives in a few months. Now they could start focusing on names and picking out baby clothes, imagining the birth of their baby girl and anticipating holding her in their waiting arms; their attention focused on my physical condition and my medical results shifted to the little miracle growing inside my belly. The news gave them the impetus and the hope they needed to begin preparing in earnest to make room for an addition to their family.

"I gave my notice at work!" Lauren announced optimistically over the phone later that week.

"Wow, Lauren, that's great!" I congratulated her.

Though I had been aware of her intentions to stop working and prepare to be a full-time mom once the surrogacy proved successful, I cheered now for her decision to follow through with that course of action. For me, her choice to stay home full-time validated the importance and life-changing momentousness of our journey through surrogacy to bring a new baby into the world.

I had witnessed signs of Henry and Lauren's growing excitement throughout the process: the joy in their voices when Dr. Wilcox confirmed the pregnancy, the squeals of delight and looks of awe at the sound of the fetal heartbeat, the wondrous curiosity of their first look at the fetal ultrasound picture, the loving and grateful acceptance of the first baby gift at Christmas. But I had worried up until now that they had not yet made any specific plans to make room for a new baby in their lives, that they had not yet engaged beyond the journey itself to their future with a child.

They had proceeded cautiously no doubt to protect themselves against possible disappointment, but with the ultrasound news of a healthy baby girl igniting their hope, they now, to my relief, appeared ready to seriously prepare to be a family. The sacrifices I had endured to be their surrogate became inconsequential footnotes when I enjoyed the pleasure of watching them finally embrace wholeheartedly this miraculous adventure and joyfully commit themselves to preparing to welcome a new life.

And with the news of a baby girl the extended families collectively stopped holding their breath. They had exhaled a sigh of relief when Dr. Wilcox had confirmed the pregnancy and my belly had begun to expand, but now they could breathe back in with excitement, preparing for a new baby girl to arrive in a few short months. This would be the first of a new generation on both sides of the family for Henry and Lauren, and now the grandparents, aunts and uncles could go out and happily fulfill their desires to buy outrageous baby outfits.

Opening the mailbox one day, I received a note from one of the grandmothers-to-be, my Aunt Pam. She had always railed against the futility of squandering time writing thank you notes, but I had written her one anyway a few weeks earlier thanking her for a Christmas gift, and now she had sent me a thank you note for my thank you note! The rules of the game had definitely changed: surrogacy had rewritten them. Aunt Pam's note proved to be a thinly concealed excuse to thank me again in writing for the journey I had chosen to take with Henry and Lauren, and I considered fully for the first time the impact of my decision, not only on my cousin and his wife but also on the people who loved them dearly. I found it deeply gratifying that my choice was enriching the lives of so many, and that I had touched my aunt deeply with my offer and the promise of a granddaughter.

With the baby now more of a reality, Henry and Lauren looked even more earnestly for any way they could help me and Robert out in thanks for choosing to grant their wish of a family.

"Why don't you guys plan a trip to get out of town, and we'll watch your kids for you," they offered one night on the phone after I had shared a pregnancy update.

The surrogacy, of course, would be traveling with us, but a change of scenery, I thought, would be entirely welcome, so in February, when I finally felt up to it, we took them up on their offer and headed to Las Vegas for a couple of days of R&R. Sharing the pregnancy had demanded a lot of energy and effort in keeping others included, and the novelty had started to wane a bit, so I found myself grateful for a few days alone with my husband, relieved for the gift of private time which had become far too scarce.

Shifting gears after a long drive from San Diego, we stepped into the *New York, New York* hotel and surveyed our surroundings, musing at the recreated NYC street scene we found ourselves suddenly cast amidst on our way to the elevator. It required only a couple of minutes in the toxic environment to remind us why we had failed to return to Las Vegas sooner. Surrounded by smokers guzzling drinks as they deposited tokens into slot machines and reset stacks of gambling chips on the tables, I found it difficult to reconcile the purposefulness of the surrogacy with the hedonistic pleasures of Vegas, and I instinctively covered my belly in an attempt to protect the life growing inside me from its negative influence.

However, I could hardly complain about a weekend away from the stresses of our daily lives, and we happily rode the elevator up to settle into our room. A giant Jacuzzi bath tub dominated the middle of the suite, a refuge in which to soak my aching pregnant body, perhaps no less gaudy an amenity, but still an infinitely more practical one than the stereotypical fantasy mirrors on the ceiling. I disrobed and climbed in the tub to unwind while Robert relaxed in front of a basketball game on the giant screen television. What can I say, the pregnancy had shifted our priorities to extracurricular activities beyond the bed.

Though making love to a wife whose belly bulged with another man's baby presented a very different context for Robert, in reality he regarded it as no more or less strange for him than with my other pregnancies. He had, in fact, cautiously limited indulging his natural instincts each time I had carried a baby, concerned with potentially jeopardizing the safety of the pregnancy (despite a lack of supporting evidence), determined to practice *safe sex* with his pregnant wife. In Robert's words: since a woman's *approach*, designed by nature to be a multiple use apparatus, appeared to him to be busy taking care of the baby, he considered sex to be inappropriate at times during my pregnancies.

"It's like if you were making dinner in the kitchen and I came in and made a peanut butter and jelly sandwich," he explained to me.

We managed to put the bed to use anyway (sans mirror), after the game and the tub soak, and we were both okay with that. PB&J rocks.

Over the course of the weekend, we searched out other highlights of Tinseltown, including the Bellagio fountain and most notably a night out at the fabulous "O" show of artistry by Cirque du Soleil. Forty-eight hours in Las Vegas proved to be our limit, though, and after several soothing soaks had pruned my pregnant body, we hightailed it out of that self-indulgent, surreal world of vacuous glitz and made our way back home, not particularly refreshed, but thankful for the opportunity it had provided for some free time alone.

After a long weekend of playing mom and dad to our kids, Henry and Lauren looked a little tired, but thankfully they had not chosen to rethink their decision about creating a family (though it may have scared them into researching some tips on parenting).

"Thanks for taking care of the kids. And for the weekend," I said gratefully.

"We had a lot of fun," Lauren assured us.

"Well, I'm sure they wore you out. The good news is when they are newborns, kids sleep a lot more and don't move around as much!" I promised them.

We loaded Henry and Lauren up with a car full of hand-me-down baby gear and clothes, giving them a start on preparing for the baby, before they left to head back up to Los Angeles. A few days later Henry called me.

"We decided after unloading all that baby stuff you gave us, that we better find a bigger house," he conceded.

They had quickly concluded that their cute little house in Manhattan Beach would not be able to accommodate the intimidating assortment of baby paraphernalia that comes with having a newborn in the 21st century. Within what seemed like days, they had sold their home and entered into escrow on a newer, more spacious house several blocks away, much more suitable for life with a newborn child. Their new home symbolized a fresh beginning after cancer and infertility, housing their hopes and dreams of building a future together as a family.

As we continued to progress through the second trimester, we stayed in close contact with each other, and I looked for ways to include them more directly in the pregnancy. Henry had told me that they were following along in the *What to Expect When You're Expecting* book, tracking the baby's progress as well as my condition, and delighted to know they were tracing our course, I sought to give them evidence that would reassure them that our pregnancy was progressing normally. I called Henry and Lauren up very late one night, shortly after they had moved into their new home.

"Could you please tell your daughter to quiet down and go to sleep, she is keeping me awake kicking up a storm!" I pleaded jokingly.

They had unfortunately not yet felt their baby kicking inside me, but I thought continued knowledge of fetal activity might capture some of the excitement of the pregnancy for them, and I enjoyed the reward of sharing those special moments. (I wanted to hear their joy, and sometimes I needed to be heardtoo: Please don't forget about me lying here with your child!) Though I had clearly woken Henry up with my late night call, I could hear a smile in his groggy voice.

"What? Okay, tell her I said to go to sleep," he chuckled softly. "Thanks for sharing, Pam," he sighed contentedly, replacing the phone on his bedside table and drifting back to sleep. Sweet dreams.

My voice on the phone woke Robert up that night too from a dazed sleep, but his initial irritation quickly diverged into bemusement when he listened in on my conversation with my cousin. I had considered sparing Robert the intrusion and getting up to make the call from the kitchen, but I knew he appreciated any opportunity to be included in the surrogacy connection with Henry and Lauren. It reminded him why we were doing this crazy thing. And because, as with all of my pregnancies, Robert felt responsible for supporting me and cheering me on, he appreciated sharing that responsibility of the surrogacy in a fun, compelling way with my cousin.

The kids delighted in opportunities to witness the movement inside my belly, often placing a hand there in hopes of feeling their baby cousin kick. And, keen on tracking the baby's development, they regarded our youth encyclopedia's depiction of the growth of a fetus as a treasured resource; nearly every day Lise would pull the well-worn book off the shelf, turning the pages one by one, until she reached the drawings of a baby developing through the nine months of pregnancy, and studying the pictures raptly.

"Which one does the baby look like right now, mommy?" she asked curiously. At 3 ½ years old, this marked her first time watching me grow round with a baby, and looking back and forth between my belly and those pictures, she marveled that a life so foreign, yet familiar, re-sided inside me.

"I can't wait to meet the baby," Kellie said, like an eager big sister, as she studied those drawings. Kellie, at 7 ½ a keen, intelligent, inquisi-tive little girl, often engaged me in conversations about the baby and the surrogacy, thinking and reasoning it all out until it became clear in her mind.

At 6 years old, Duncan had proven to be a typical rambunctious little boy, but he also had a sensitive, caring side to balance his full-speed-ahead boyishness, and when kicking a soccer ball or zooming his matchbox cars down the halls of the house for hours, he would sud-denly stop to run and surprise me with a hug and a kiss for my belly.

Once the kids discovered that the baby had developed enough to hear sounds coming from outside the womb, they would take turns talking to her, telling her stories, and singing her songs too.

"I love you baby," Duncan whispered into my belly.

I watched them in awe in those intimate, heartwarming moments as I witnessed their love for a cousin they had yet to meet. They acted so proud of her, their baby cousin, that you would have thought they had personally assisted Dr. Tran in transferring those embryos into my uterus. All three of our children had, in fact, accepted integral roles in this pregnancy; the surrogacy shaped their day-to-day lives and influenced their thoughts and behavior, and for their part they just could not wait to make her acquaintance.

Robert felt connected to the baby too, but his connection ran through me; he chose consciously not to engage the baby directly because he believed that privilege belonged to Henry, the baby's father. Robert's thoughts diverged on to a different path with this pregnancy; instead of making plans for the baby's future, he found himself simply admiring the intimate relationship between a pregnant woman's body and the baby inside, ever more remarkable in light of the surrogacy. His admiration for my generosity and courage in acting as a surrogate strengthened our own intimate bond. His caring and love for me deepened.

Robert bragged proudly about the surrogacy, sharing his excitement in helping Henry and Lauren realize the dream of a family with friends and acquaintances, refueled by the encouraging responses from those he trusted and respected. He loved to break the news to people with his own special sense of humor, and when his closest childhood friend, Eric, called him up one day, Robert could not resist toying with him.

"Hey, what's goin' on?" Eric asked.

"Well, Pam is pregnant again, but the baby is not mine," Robert offered, deadpan. No explanation. No response. After a long, agonizing silence, in which Eric searched in vain for a way to comfort his friend in the face of his wife's illicit wanderings, Robert added, "But it's okay because it's not hers either."

"What???" Eric barely managed to say, confused and struck speechless. Robert laughed mercilessly and then enlightened Eric with the details of our surrogacy, delighting in the opportunity to get an old friend good, and relishing the chance to blow him away with our story.

We shared news of the surrogacy every day, with updates to friends and new briefings for acquaintances, as my belly grew noticeably bigger in the second trimester, stretching against my clothing like a mound of dough rising gently against the sides of a bowl. The remodeling of my body was a visible daily reminder of the pregnancy to those around me.

The kids delivered the most memorable briefings, fresh with their own unique perspective. One weekday afternoon while Duncan shot hoops in the driveway with another boy from the neighborhood, I overheard them talking about my pregnancy through the kitchen window. Above the rhythmic dribbling of the ball against the pavement, I could hear bits and pieces of Duncan's explanation to his friend.

"My baby cousin is growing inside my Mom…(bounce, bounce)……. the baby's mom can't carry her…(bounce, bounce)…. my mom will give her back when she comes out…… (swish)…..," he explained.

I strained to hear more, but lost the conversation in the commotion of the game, and soon they had moved onto a new topic. I chuckled at how the two young boys had easily shared the intricacies of embryo transfer in a few words between baskets, unaware or maybe just unconcerned about its complex nature, accepting at face value the role of surrogacy simply as a different way of bringing a baby into the world.

Children as a rule appeared much less concerned than the adults with whom we shared the surrogacy. I had fun delivering the news too, though adults predictably responded less matter-of-factly, typically with raised eyebrows and a confused, shocked expression. However, more often than not such an encounter would evolve from an awkward silence into a hug and share fest, often with virtual strangers, prompting public displays of affection that would have left my father-in-law blushing.

Endorsements from friends and family who admired my choice to make a sacrifice to help a couple bring new life into the world provided me with much needed boosts of encouragement along the way. Robert's Aunt Joan penned me a sweet note: *I am in awe of your love of others, courage and tenacity…..we're all very proud of you*, she wrote. And I beamed at his Aunt Jane's reaction, when we bumped into her dining out one night at a local restaurant: she jumped up from her seat and threw her arms around me, proceeding to regale her dinner companions with my story, her eyes twinkling with delight (theirs, on the other hand, twinkled with quiet shock).

I tried not to be disappointed on the rare occasions when a distant family member or acquaintance declined to enthusiastically embrace my decision for personal or religious reasons, but I found it difficult to understand how people could claim that the quest I had embarked upon could be considered *wrong* or *unnatural* when it precipitated so much natural, unadulterated joy in others. In the end I simply chose to focus on the positive responses of the people I admired and respected.

Some women upon hearing my story would respond enthusiastically, "*I would do that!*", and while they all may have sincerely believed that, I think only a few of them would have actually followed through on it. Given the array of mental and physical challenges I had already personally experienced, I believed it took a certain type of person to follow through successfully on a surrogacy, and I advised any woman considering taking the journey to conduct some serious soul searching before making a concrete offer that goes beyond a gut reaction or a guilt check. While I harbored no regrets about my own experience, surrogacy had irrefutably altered my life over the last year and that of those around me who I loved dearly. Surrogacy so far had been a great, positive, transforming kind of adventure, but without the right frame of mind, approach and family support I imagined it could potentially have been an unmitigated disaster.

Over the past year I had discovered the key ingredients in a successful approach to surrogacy to be *honesty* and *trust* with both myself and my husband, as well as with Henry and Lauren. In the beginning

I had found it crucial to be honest with myself about my true desire to become a surrogate, for if that desire had proven shallow and insincere or selfish and false, I would have quickly regretted my decision, resenting the sacrifices I had made and without the mental strength to face the inherent challenges. And I had needed to trust myself from the start, trust my strength and capabilities to be able to gracefully (or at least readily) handle the unknown challenges that presented themselves along the way.

Honesty in my relationship with my husband had also proven to be imperative, specifically both his honesty with me about his willingness to support and share the surrogacy and his openness about his concerns, without which there might have festered a minefield of potential resentment and bitterness in our relationship. Like me, thankfully, he had viewed our choice to pursue the surrogacy as a sacred, immutable promise to Henry and Lauren, and he had accepted the need to relegate romance to the back burner, to cater to me when I felt sick and to take over for me when I was tired, without harboring any resentments or regrets, because those inconveniences were easily absorbed and forgotten in light of our lofty goal. I had needed also to trust in Robert, my partner, to always be there for me when the doubts and fears and frustrations inevitably crept in. I knew going in to the surrogacy that I could trust him to pick me back up, and he had certainly been there to make the surrogacy easier for me by not only physically performing tasks, but also encouraging me during the difficult times.

When I had felt sick and defeated by nausea for a couple of months and the reality of the long road of surrogacy had settled in, Robert had allowed me to vent without judgment, then carefully and gingerly brought me back to the purpose and fun of our wondrous adventure with Henry and Lauren, inspiring me to push forward with a positive frame of mind. Knowing intuitively that surrogacy required me to give so deeply, he considered it his duty to ensure I received as well, giving to me whatever he could at every opportunity. And I had trusted him to be there for me like that.

Finally, honesty with Henry and Lauren, the intended parents, had proven to be the foundation of a satisfying surrogacy, though admittedly it was not always easy to be honest with emotions running high and deep. I had sometimes found it difficult to tell them when I had felt frustrated with the whole surrogacy in the midst of a severe hormone-induced nausea in the first few months, or when I had been concerned that they had not yet embraced the surrogacy in the 5th month, or when I had wished on occasion that I could hide the pregnancy and just be me. I refrained, in fact, from telling them everything I thought and felt, because I had no interest in scaring them unnecessarily, but I had learned the importance of creating an open line of communication about feelings, needs and desires, allowing all of us to feel linked, understood, and appreciated.

And the trust in our relationship had enabled us to share the intimacies of the journey: the wonder of the baby's heartbeat and movement, our personal hopes and expectations, the joy of preparing for a family. Without the ability to share those experiences, the surrogacy would have become a hollow adventure.

While my venture as a surrogate touched many of my friends and acquaintances, my willingness to make sacrifices to deliver Henry and Lauren a child most deeply affected those who had faced issues of infertility in their struggle to have children; it gave them a chance to hope and dream. Several cancer survivors took comfort in hearing my quest as a source of positive focus amidst a devastating cycle of illness.

One morning retrieving the newspaper from outside on the driveway, I stopped to talk to our neighbor, Diane, the nurse, a cancer survivor (a few times over). Like many people I have met who have looked death squarely in the eye, I admired Diane's honesty and forthrightness, and her realness. She stopped me and laid her hand purposefully on my arm, holding my eyes intently in hers.

"I think what you are doing is really amazing and I wanted you to know that," Diane said simply, before she walked away.

Because cancer and treatment had stripped her of the possibility of children, she knew the personal devastation of infertility. I walked back into the house, paper in hand, tears clouding my vision.

Lauren embraced the opportunity around this time to share the story of our surrogacy at a "celebration of life" picnic with other cancer patient survivors from the center in Los Angeles where doctors had treated her, bringing a story of hope and possibility to many women and families there who had suffered through the indignities of cancer. Sharing our surrogacy adventure seemed to have a way of healing or at least mitigating the pain of others who had suffered through infertility and illness, and inspired some others, I hope, to at least consider the power of that kind of giving.

We concluded the second trimester around Valentine's Day, when Lauren and Henry sent me an unexpected gift of new maternity clothes. That bright surprise that landed on my doorstep served to diffuse in an instant the frustrations of the boredom and weariness that had visited me recently, after six long months of pregnancy.

Trying on the comfy cute overalls and soft stretchy sweats that added welcome variety to my limited wardrobe, I luxuriated in their flattering fit and fresh feel which would serve me well into the coming final trimester. Though chocolate and flowers may be the more typical gift in recognition of the holiday devoted to *love*, my new clothes recognized in a fitting way Henry and Lauren's love and appreciation for the gift I held safely in my womb. I smiled inwardly at the thrill evident in their words written on the note inside the package.

"We're so excited……..3 months away!" it said. And so it was.

THE THIRD TRIMESTER

The Baby is Coming!

AT SIX MONTHS PREGNANT I slipped into the last trimester, my belly resembling a ripe melon under the fitted contours of my maternity clothing. Every week that passed by as we progressed closer to *the big day*, the focus of my daily thoughts and interactions shifted with gathering excitement to the surrogate baby inside me.

Thoughts of their baby girl filled Henry and Lauren's waking hours too, as they prepared for her arrival, transforming the baby's room into a bright cheery garden with a custom paint job meticulously executed by Henry. Shopping for a crib, a sturdy stroller and a trustworthy car seat, he thoroughly researched the safety and quality records of each item purchased, passionately embracing the mission of the prudent expectant father.

The expectation and joy of the grandparents increased dramatically as well, as we advanced closer to a due date, and at the end of February the postman delivered a surprise package on my doorstep from Lauren's parents. Slitting open the carefully packaged box marked

FRAGILE, I found a card on top proclaiming, *"Joy!"* on its cover with the printed message, *"What a joy it is to welcome this precious new life."* Inside Joyce had penned a heartfelt note that said, *"Thank you for making this dream a reality! You have truly given a selfless gift of love.......We are here for you always."* Under the note and a mound of white Styrofoam peanuts I discovered a lovely Lladro porcelain figurine of a young girl in a wide-brimmed hat, cradling an apron-full of spring flowers, long neatly plaited braids spilling down the front of her dress.

I delighted in this unexpected gift of love and appreciation from Joyce and Jerry, a delicate tribute to the innocence and preciousness of a little girl, reveling in their joy at the gift of a granddaughter, and in their promise to be *here for you always.* Those powerful words assured me that they would not discard their appreciation for me after the birth of the baby, but remember forever my gift to all of them.

I had begun in recent weeks to worry about the emptiness I would suffer when the surrogacy ended; emptiness triggered not by the absence of a baby in my house, but the result of the abrupt ending of the unique and special status I had grown accustomed to over the last several months as a surrogate mom for Henry and Lauren. After a year traveling on an all-consuming journey, how would I be able to adjust back to reality, to *normal*? Would I want to? And would *normal* look the same any more?

Gazing at the wistful expression on that porcelain figurine, I paused to imagine how the baby inside of me would look as a young girl, how her personality and appearance would develop over the coming years. Would she grow up to wear her hair in long braids and pick flowers for the secret joy of admiring their simple beauty? Or race down the mountain at Squaw Valley without fear like her daredevil father, skis flying over the fresh snow? Would she sport Henry's wide smile or Lauren's engaging sense of humor? Love to read Nancy Drew mysteries? Change the course of someone's life?

Though her life pulsed spiritedly inside me, I could not divine her destiny, but only hope to watch from a distance as she grew into her precious uniqueness, defining her own place in the world over the coming years. I did not expect or hope to be integrally involved in her day to day life, but I treasured the promise of the opportunity to watch her future unfold, her personality develop, her dreams pursued; without taking any credit for whom she becomes, I could be proud of giving her life.

On March 8th, Lauren and I walked in for our seven month appointment with Dr. Gerber to check on the status of that infant girl tumbling around inside of me. We sat down and chatted amiably in the waiting room, surrounded by several other women, some visibly pregnant and others not. As I glanced around the office between bits of our conversation, I observed furtive looks in our direction; a flurry of attention shifting to my swollen belly, with curiosity, scrutiny and disdain hanging heavily in the air between us. Through my fog of confusion, suddenly a realization hit me upside the head: those women had mistaken Lauren and me for a lesbian couple. (*Not that there is anything wrong with that*, except that it characterized our relationship in a sweeping misrepresentation). When the nurse called us in to the exam room to wait for Dr. Gerber, I turned to Lauren as soon as the door closed behind us.

"Did you see those women looking at us? I think they thought we were a lesbian couple!" I whispered in shocked revelation.

"I was thinking the same thing!" Lauren cried in disbelief.

A moment we had not anticipated, we laughed about it self-consciously at first, and then simply cracked up at the absurdity of the idea, though we could not necessarily fault them for coming to that false conclusion, given the circumstances.

That encounter did make me think, though. I have friends who are gay and I believe in the right of gay people to be parents, but would

I have offered to carry this baby for a gay couple? I do not think I can answer that question honestly without having faced it head-on in reality, but I know it would have been a more complicated decision for me. I had offered to be a surrogate for my cousin, because cancer had robbed his wife of the ability to carry a child, restoring to them a privilege that had been taken away. If my cousin were in a homosexual relationship, I may have been less compelled to sacrifice for a fundamentally different situation, in which I would be introducing them to the possibility of a new privilege that had never been theirs to begin with; though just because they never could have carried a baby, does not mean they would have longed for a child of their own any less. Loving my cousin, no matter what, I know I would have considered it, but I simply cannot know how I would have ultimately responded. Many women who contract with surrogacy agencies do opt to carry children for gay couples.

Back in Dr. Gerber's office three weeks later on March 28th for my next routine appointment, this time an entourage accompanied me into the waiting room. In addition to Lauren and her mom, Joyce, Robert joined me for our visit along with Kellie, Duncan, and Lise. When the nurse assistant called my name that morning, SEVEN of us stood up and marched down the hallway, like a posse of Snow White's dwarves, crowding into an exam room together to wait for Dr. Gerber en masse.

That afternoon marked the only time the kids accompanied us to an OB appointment, because not only did it prove easier to go while they were in school, but also because I felt those doctor visits should remain personal and private for Lauren, paralleling as much as possible the normal circumstances for a new mother-to-be. Robert typically stayed away of his own accord for the same reasons, not feeling like it was his place to be there, not wanting to crowd in on Lauren and Henry's space. Often without Henry able to leave work, Lauren and

I enjoyed the time alone together on those doctor visits to bond as mothers in partnership; but not that morning.

Smiling and admirably poised as she maneuvered her way into the room past everyone, Dr. Gerber greeted us all warmly and then focused on the business at hand; monitoring the baby's heartbeat, measuring fundus height, and checking my blood pressure, while the onlookers attempted unsuccessfully to fade into the corners of that tiny room. If she had not fully appreciated the reality of the group effort to bring this baby into the world before, our appearance that morning spelled out in clear view the complex intricacies of a surrogacy relationship. Dr. Gerber appeared delighted that morning to be party to the unique dynamics of this unusual pregnancy.

Completing her checks, she declared the baby and pregnancy normal, reassuring us with the news that we had successfully reached the magic 32 week marker of the pregnancy. Should an early emergency delivery be required, the newborn would be able to breathe outside the womb on her own; the relief and excitement at having reached that milestone permeated the room. The probability of delivering a healthy baby to Henry and Lauren stood now firmly in our favor, and we walked out of that room together with smiles on our faces, giddy at the success of our surrogacy and giggly at the impact our entourage made at the doctor's office that morning. There were more than a few surprised stares when all seven of us filed back triumphantly through the waiting room and out the door, like the dwarves after a successful foray into the forest. *Hi, Ho!*

Though Robert only made an appearance at a couple of my obstetrical appointments in addition to the one that morning, that record of attendance belied his excitement about the surrogacy. He continued to share our adventure with his friends and colleagues into this third trimester, delighting as always in surreptitiously shocking them with the news.

One night a couple months shy of our due date, at a trade show conference dinner with some newly acquainted business colleagues, he answered some seemingly innocuous questions about the details of his family life over dinner, familiarizing his table companions with me and our three children.

"And my wife is pregnant!" he announced proudly. His colleagues shouted congratulations up and down the dinner table, until a quiet pause hung briefly like an exhaled breath over the gathering.

"But this one's not mine," Robert added dramatically, an impermeable, stony expression on his face.

The conversation and congratulations stopped dead. He hesitated a minute while this group of people who were barely familiar with him or his warped sense of humor agonized over how to respond, before he stepped back in with impeccable timing to follow up.

"It's o.k., though, because it's not hers either," he offered.

Robert's fascination with making people squirm with anticipation before hitting them squarely in the eye with the punch line often causes me to wonder whether he missed a calling as a stand-up comedian. Confused and uncomfortable pursuing the story further that night, Robert's table companions quietly shifted the conversation to a different topic. Not until the following morning, after many inquiring guesses, did he share with them the story of our surrogacy.

When he recited this incident to me later that week, he delighted in the impact of his sneaky humorous delivery, yet also mused over the emotional connection he made that night with colleagues who barely knew him. He marveled at their urge to embrace him the next day like long lost friends, their faces flushed with emotion after hearing about the surrogacy. Always one to appreciate the benefits of a good hug, Robert reveled in the random hugging that is par for the course with surrogacy, and he basked in the admiration and appreciation for his part in helping make our journey through surrogacy succeed.

In this last trimester, increasingly often my obviously protruding belly inevitably forced me to explain the surrogacy to people with whom I might rather not wish to share those intimate details. Though the sight of my belly made the pregnancy public, I regarded surrogacy as a personal journey, and after the novelty of explaining the surrogacy wore off, often I would prefer to guard our story protectively and share it only with those for whom it would have real meaning. When strangers congratulated me on the baby and asked me questions like *"what number will this be"?*, often I would answer vaguely to avoid having to uncover the details of the surrogacy relationship. But sometimes it became unavoidable, and one day, picking up some pictures at the local photo shop with my three children in tow, the store owner noticed my pregnancy.

"With another baby you'll have four kids!" he pointed out bluntly, an incredulous tone in his voice.

"Yep," I remarked (untruthfully), attempting to move past his remarks. But he continued to question me about my decision to have a fourth child, and so I finally explained to him the truth.

"Well, it's really not mine, I'm just carrying it for someone else," I said, with as much matter-of-fact finality in my voice as I could muster.

"Hey, you can make a lot of money doing that!" he responded indiscreetly, before I could escape from the store with my pictures in hand. Oh, boy. Standing there, almost eight months pregnant, feeling tired, heavy, awkward and getting anxious for the pregnancy to end, the crass remark set me off seething, and I wanted to yell back to him: "Would **you** do this just for the money??!!!!!"

"While I am not actually getting paid to *do that*, because I am carrying this child for my cousin, money is actually not the priority of any surrogate," I countered instead, controlling my voice in a foolish attempt to educate him. "There are substantial sacrifices surrogates make that a wad of money could never repay," I lectured him. But he failed to hear me, unwilling or unable to believe in the inherent value of giving that is the primary motivation of surrogates, and so I am afraid my pointed diatribe failed to enlighten him. It proved best sometimes, I learned, to just keep my mouth shut and smile.

However, I did wish a few days later that I **had** opened my mouth and blabbered to a stranger, when a cop stopped me as I raced to get the kids to school on time. He peered in the car window and asked for my license and registration without noticing my feet swollen in my slippers, my belly bumping up against the steering wheel, or the exhaustion written across my face.

"Are you serious? Look at me!" I wanted to yell at him. I wonder if I'd had the presence of mind at that moment to tell him my story of surrogacy, if he would have been inclined to reward my good deed with a decision not to write me up for a ticket. Ah, well, probably not.

On April 3rd, about six weeks before the May 22nd estimated delivery date, my children presented me with a gift for my 36th birthday when I woke up lazily in bed that morning.

"Happy Birthday, Mommy," Lise and Kellie and Duncan whispered to me. Inside the lovingly wrapped and haphazardly taped together package, I uncovered a soft knitted blanket the kids had chosen together as the perfect present for me.

"You just seem to really like to nap," Kellie explained, proud of the choice they had made.

And in that moment I realized, with a pang of guilt, that from their perspective I often appeared tired, disinclined to play catch, bake cookies, or play a game together. Over the last seven and a half months I had failed to be as readily available to Kellie, Duncan or Lise, a sacrifice they were forced to endure in an effort to bring a family to Henry and Lauren. And saddened by my failure, I wondered, *was this fair to them?* I vowed to do better. The kids seldom complained, though, and more often than not responded with sympathy and understanding, embracing their sacrifices readily to help their new cousin into the world. And so, upon receiving that poignantly appropriate birthday present, mixed with some regret over their loss, I felt lucky and proud of my three small children.

Although Robert flew out of town on business later that morning of my birthday, Lauren arrived to treat me to a mini-vacation at the luxurious four-star Aviara Resort in nearby Carlsbad to continue my celebration. After an elegant lunch together, Lauren drove off on her own to retrieve all three of my children from school, while I enjoyed the pleasure of indulging myself like a pampered princess in the spa at the Resort for an afternoon, with a gift of a birthday massage from Henry and Lauren.

I walked out of the doors of the Aviara refreshed and relaxed, returning home to a houseful of joyful organized activity Lauren had prepared to entertain the kids for the afternoon. They always looked forward to the visits from Lauren and Henry, happily welcoming them into their lives, sharing stories from school, taking their hands to show them a new beloved book or stuffed animal, drawing them into our family fold. While Lauren engaged them, I sinfully rested quietly with a magazine. My own nanny for the day!

The birthday card Lauren gave me that afternoon said: *"I bet you never would have thought that at thirty-six you'd be pregnant with someone else's baby!"* Nope, I never would have seen that one coming; had not even known the possibility existed. It sounded like a tabloid headline. The truth is I do not even like being pregnant all that much, but now I found myself unable to imagine the past year without taking this journey.

It is always hard to envision what the future may hold, and quite honestly I prefer it that way, watching the magic of life unfold as I live it, rather than plotting its course like a flight plan. At eighteen I would have probably considered doubling my age to thirty-six practically dead, the fun and excitement of life a distant memory. Ha! I had learned in the intervening years that though the nature of the adventures in my thirty's may be different from backpacking through Europe in my twenty's, the excitement of life never waned. It is all in the approach.

And now, entering what people disdainfully refer to as *middle age*, I found myself living life not as a boring old housewife settled into a predetermined routine, but as somewhat of a risk-taking renegade inviting new and daring experiences into my repertoire of achievements. (Well, don't let me get carried away with myself. Amelia Earhart I am not; my feet remained firmly planted on the ground, even though I might not currently be able to see them.) *"Wow what a year it's been"* Lauren wrote in closing on the card. Wow, indeed.

I reveled in my favored status as the birthday girl that day, loved, and admired by my family, and appreciated for my special role as surrogate mother for Lauren and Henry's baby. As the birthdays had piled up after my 30th, the gifts meant less to me, and the ridiculous number of candles on my cake had become more of an invitation to scrutinize what I had achieved in my life. This year, though, I could take pride in a tangible, remarkable accomplishment, and the number itself no longer carried such ominous weight.

Lauren, clearly intent on taking special care of me and showing me yet again her deep appreciation, had thoughtfully arranged to treat me to a special birthday dinner with the kids that evening at my favorite seafood restaurant in Del Mar, where my sister, Heidi, joined all of us to dabble in delicious delicacies. That night, surrounded by family and placed seemingly up on a pedestal at an elevated table with an ocean view, I felt honored for my courage and compassion. Instead of an ordinary birthday, I found myself celebrating a more profound life event, borrowing against my birthday and my life for the life and future birthdays of the unborn baby inside me.

Lauren chauffeured us home after I blew out the candles on my dessert, and as I settled my weary, lopsided self into a pile of pillows on my bed later that night, the fatigue of the final stretch of the pregnancy overtaking me, I drifted off smiling at the cherished care and generosity Lauren had bestowed upon me. An unusual, but treasured, birthday passed.

A few days later, amidst a couple of late birthday cards, I found a letter from the courts informing us Robert and I were being "sued" by Lauren and Henry for establishment of parentage of the child in my womb. Oh, great, some more warm and fuzzy surrogacy legal rhetoric. While we were eager to sign the papers the California courts required to give Henry and Lauren their deserved legal recognition as parents, it proved a bit disconcerting to be the "defendants" in a lawsuit brought on by my cousin. But we all derived comfort from a binding written legal agreement, and whatever process satisfied the courts pleased us as well if it assured that everyone recognized that the baby inside of me belonged only to Henry and Lauren, forever theirs to keep and care for as the rightful parents.

Parental establishment, now legal and final, necessitated another legal action, namely that Henry and Lauren draft a will or living trust that included their baby-to-be and specifically designated their desires for her care and well-being should they perish. While I realized the odds on that scenario were rather far-fetched, I found it reassuring that Henry and Lauren would have in place a future for their baby girl should they no longer be available to care for her. My sense of responsibility dictated I ensure a secure future for the baby I helped bring into the world before I handed her over, and while I had always been confident that Henry and Lauren would be wonderful parents, the will provided for her should they not be there to carry out that life-long responsibility, as morbid as that may be to consider, providing me an added measure of peace of mind.

Having surmounted, I hoped, all of the major legal challenges of a surrogacy arrangement, as well as the medical challenges of a surrogate pregnancy, the last month before the birth could focus solely on me and the baby. In that final month my calls with Henry and Lauren became more frequent and took on an added sense of anticipation and excitement, our conversations more animated each day.

"Are you guys getting excited?" I asked repeatedly in those final weeks.

"We are so excited! I can't believe it's almost time," Lauren's voice echoed back to me. The checkered flag had appeared and we were racing barely in control of our escalating giddiness to the finish line.

Henry called me occasionally from his office in downtown L.A. in the middle of the workday to check in on me, and I loved that his excitement for this baby I carried distracted him from the mountain of work screaming for his attention. The controlled jubilance in his voice often took me back to that moment when I had decided to offer to be a surrogate so he could be a father, and, as I had dared hope, this journey we had chosen to take together had succeeded from the very beginning in creating a special bond that linked us forever. And while his excitement in the final weeks obviously focused on the baby, he never stopped caring about me and my state of physical and mental health, not just because I carried his child around inside, but because he appreciated so dearly that I had chosen to take that journey in a loving effort to give him a family.

Late in April, amidst the feverish last few weeks of the surrogacy, Robert and I were invited to attend a wedding shower for my college friend, Stacey, and her fiancé at the home of my friend, Maureen, in Los Angeles. Though thrilled about the opportunity to visit with good friends, I felt as huge and ungainly as a beached hippo at this point in the pregnancy, and wearing some matronly maternity dress at a party where all of my friends would undoubtedly more closely simulate gracefully glamorous Hollywood screen stars, failed to thrill me.

As had been the case carrying my own babies, I became increasingly anxious in the last month for the pregnancy to come to an end, to be back inside my old self, and there were some days I wished I could just step out of the pregnancy for a day or two, a temporary reprieve from feeling awkward, exhausted and overwhelmingly less than glamorous.

As the night of the party approached I searched the maternity stores in every corner of San Diego County in vain for a number that would reveal the soft glow of pregnancy while simultaneously hinting at my hidden inner sex goddess. And my husband thinks I ask too much from one little dress!

The evening of the party I wriggled my way into an appealing, soft print maternity dress a friend had loaned me earlier that week, and put myself together as best I could. With the emotional ups and downs of pregnancy, and my anticipation about the evening ahead, I felt a bit on edge when I took a look in the mirror, and discovered to my disappointment the overall effect below my lofty expectations. Just at that moment, before my frustrations could take hold of me, all three of my precious children tiptoed into my bedroom.

"You look really pretty, Mommy," they declared affectionately, looking me over closely from the mascara on my eyelashes to the curves of my dress to my high heel shoes.

Their adoration trumped my disappointment, and so the dress managed to live up to my hopes that night, even if, as I suspect, Robert is the one who put the kids up to it; he had become adept at anticipating my pregnancy-induced fragile emotional states, and always sought subtle ways to boost my spirits and pre-empt any hormonal meltdowns, for my sake and his too. I understood more clearly that night the truth that half of the secret to looking beautiful or sexy is a projection of how you feel inside, and at the party the compliments I received were a reflection of the pride I had discovered in my children's admiring comments.

A couple of days later on April 24th Robert and I met Henry and Lauren at Dr. Gerber's office. Though Lauren and I had visited Dr. Gerber just two weeks earlier for a routine exam, now that the pregnancy had advanced closer to term the doctor wanted to monitor the baby's progress more frequently. And Robert and Henry joined us that morning too, so that we could discuss the upcoming due date together and make a group decision on scheduling the delivery and designing the final preparations for the big day. We had joined together a year ago in this amazing journey through surrogacy, and we all wanted the important decisions we made about the day of delivery to be agreed upon as a team, in support of one another, to ensure the most meaningful, successful culminating moment of all our hopes and efforts.

Together with Dr. Gerber we had decided early on in the pregnancy that the safest and most responsible route would be to proceed with a scheduled c-section. While I would have preferred not to deliver the baby inside me surgically, we were all weary of the risks, based on my previous deliveries, of yet another baby becoming wedged precariously inside my womb during the birth process. I shared with Robert my secret hope, though, that if perhaps I went into labor early I could deliver the baby naturally, but, worried about another traumatic delivery and fearful of the mortal risk to me, he strongly voiced his support to stick with a c-section no matter when I delivered.

Though I understand that a cesarean section is a safe alternative birthing method, delivering Kellie by c-section had left me with a temporary sense of disappointment and failure seven years earlier. In a term paper I found recently that I had written for my university Human Biology class on the effects of cesarean section births on the mother, research about the origin of those negative feelings pointed to a perception of a loss of control at the birth, a perception I recalled all too vividly from the frightening emergency intervention required with Kellie. I had never imagined when I wrote that paper at Stanford that seven years later I, myself, would turn out to be one of those women compelled to submit to a c-section. I had firmly believed that my tough, fit, gymnastics body could handle a natural delivery effortlessly, and for god sakes women had given birth successfully for thousands and thousands of years.

I struggled with acute feelings of inadequacy when my body could not pull through a natural delivery with Kellie, but in hindsight if I had given birth thousands of years earlier without the option of a c-section, Kellie and I would likely have appeared as mortality statistics in the annual census. Surviving by c-section proved an infinitely more palatable alternative. And I comforted myself with the knowledge that, though I viewed a c-section as a procedure to be endured in lieu of the transcendently beautiful experience of a natural delivery, planning a scheduled c-section would give me a measure of control, hopefully providing me with a more positive birth experience than the emergency delivery of Kellie.

I reminded myself that this birth event first and foremost would be for the benefit and consideration of another couple, the baby's parents, whose own sense of control had spiraled away from them when they first heard the word "*cancer*". As Robert pointed out to me, Henry and Lauren arguably deserved any measure of assurance and safety we could provide them; this was, after all, their baby. And planning a c-section allowed Henry and Lauren the opportunity to prepare mentally and logistically for a specific date when they could be sure to be present in the operating room. Though the planning of the birth event inevitably steals some of the mystery and wonder from the birth itself, it is also true that a surrogacy birth, whether by surgical or natural delivery, represents a wondrous miracle all its own.

And so, on Dr. Gerber's recommendation, we chose Monday, May 14th, the Monday after Mother's Day, as our scheduled c-section delivery date, eight days before the estimated due date of May 22nd. Able to focus on an actual date now when they would become parents, when they could welcome their daughter into the world, Henry and Lauren could circle that date in red on the calendar and hold onto another real and concrete piece of evidence that their dream would really be coming true. And soon! The finish line was coming up rapidly to meet us; in three weeks we would cut the cord that attached all of us together.

After meeting with Dr. Gerber that morning, we drove over to Scripps Memorial Hospital in Encinitas for a brief tour of the location and surroundings where the baby would be born. We pre-registered with some paperwork, visited the labor rooms, and peeked into the operating room and the recovery rooms, where we would all be thrown together for the baby's scheduled entrance into the world. The tour introduced Henry and Lauren to the ins and outs of a hospital maternity ward, and together allowed all four of us the opportunity to visualize and familiarize ourselves with the environment for our surrogate delivery.

"Well, this is where we will be. It feels a little bit different from where we delivered Kellie, Duncan and Lise, but it looks nice," I observed.

"I can't believe we are actually going to walk in here in a few weeks to have a baby," Lauren marveled.

Walking around the halls of that hospital so near the delivery date, we could imagine, for the first time, the impending birth as a tangible reality. Our hearts pumping rapidly with exhilaration, we practically skipped out the hospital doors after our tour ended, though my awkward belly prevented any entertainment of that motion in the literal sense.

"Oh my gosh! This is actually happening!" Lauren gushed, grinning broadly.

From the hospital we climbed back in our cars and drove up the freeway to Carlsbad, to meet again with our psychologist, Karen Chernekoff, for lunch at a local restaurant. She had requested to meet with us for lunch that afternoon to develop a plan to guide the integral decisions for the day of the birth, advising us that emotions run high in the midst of that momentous event.

We reflected with Karen on the success of our quest together over the last year since we had first met to evaluate the viability of a surrogacy relationship among us, and she congratulated all of us on a surrogacy that had played out so beautifully.

"I wish all of my couples could have experiences like you," she said.

While she acknowledged that we had been lucky to navigate the medical maze of surrogacy so smoothly, Karen appeared most heartened by the understanding and empathy we had for each other which had allowed us to embrace the journey together without some of the typical misunderstandings and complications that can clutter the surrogacy landscape.

We discussed that afternoon the specific logistical details of a birth plan to guide the hospital delivery, in an effort to clarify a vision for the birth and hospital stay that would serve all our needs and desires in a mutually satisfying design. Karen had already spoken to the staff at the hospital to apprise them of our surrogacy relationship, and reported back to us that ours would be the first surrogate delivery at that hospital. Because they had never handled a surrogate birth, the hospital staff had responded with understandable concern about the logistics and emotions surrounding this unusual event, and thus, a well thought out and detailed birth plan would prove invaluable to them as well.

"So, are you planning on all of you being there for the delivery?" she asked.

"Yes, definitely," we all answered together, agreeing that all four of us should be able to be present at the hospital and in the operating room for the birth on May 14th.

"There's no way I'm doing this without all of us in that delivery room," I insisted.

While my presence would be a foregone conclusion, the presence of the other three in that operating room would be of tantamount importance to me, and quite frankly not negotiable. Henry and Lauren deserved the opportunity to witness their daughter's birth, and without them in attendance the birth would feel like a woefully incomplete and inadequate celebration, like a cake without frosting, or more pertinently like frosting without a cake, nothing to hold it up, and nothing to give it substance. And though Robert's presence at the birth would not be essential for delivery, his presence by my side would be essential to my peace of mind. I counted on his support and care on an undoubtedly physically and emotionally trying day for me, and without him there I would feel very much alone, knowing that Henry and Lauren would be understandably focused on the baby. I had envisioned that day of the birth from the minute I had decided to offer to be a surrogate, and Robert had always been there standing beside me in that picture. Without him there would be like having your best friend coach you through the season to the championship and then fail to show up for the final.

Perhaps the most sensitive issue unique to a surrogate birth that we discussed with Karen that afternoon regarded who would hold the baby first.

"The baby should definitely be given to Henry and Lauren first. No question," I answered quickly. "But if you guys wouldn't mind, I'd love to hold her soon afterward," I requested tentatively.

"Absolutely, Pam," Henry answered.

While I believe that Henry and Lauren would have deferred to me if I had indicated a fervent wish to hold the baby right away, to their unspoken relief I responded immediately and adamantly that, as the parents, they should absolutely embrace their child first. But I asked their permission for a chance to hold the baby too in those first few minutes, so I could welcome her into the world and witness for myself her healthy and whole perfection, clasping her warm little body against mine after nurturing her inside me. Fearing my request might worry Henry and Lauren about me bonding with the baby, I had struggled with the decision to request that privilege, but they were thankfully unhesitating about granting that wish. I failed to feel in any way feel like the baby's mother, but I anticipated an instinctive maternal desire to share a moment with her in the space outside of my womb, to acknowledge and appreciate our connection over the last nine months, to see her, touch her, breathe her in before her world widened considerably.

"And what about in recovery, after the baby is born, how do you envision that time?" Karen asked.

"We all want to be able to be together in the hospital recovery room after she is born, and I want Lauren to be able to sleep in the room with us," I insisted.

"The hospital won't be able to guarantee you a private room, but I'll make sure to request that you can all be together in recovery," she reassured us.

We shared a mutual desire that for the two to three day recovery following our c-section birth, the baby and Mom and me could all stay together in a private hospital room, and that all four of us be issued identifying tags that allowed us to be alone with her there. The opportunity to watch Henry and Lauren bond with their baby, cuddling and caring for her, connecting together as a family, would provide me reassurance and reward for my sacrifices over the last year. Though I worried that it might be awkward at times for all of us to share that space together, that vision of family bonding and connection is what I had held dear for the last nine months, the one that pulled me through the shots, nausea and fatigue, the one that made it all worthwhile.

Because it is highly unusual to have four parents in the delivery room or more than one mother in the recovery room (go figure), Karen would be responsible for communicating our wishes to the hospital and ironing out any concerns or questions beforehand to ensure our vision of the birth would come to fruition. She composed a letter which she delivered to the hospital a few days before the scheduled delivery, outlining our wishes, and assuring their staff that Henry, Lauren, Robert and I were *"....respective of one another and mutually enthusiastic about the upcoming birth......this is a wonderful circumstance of family helping family overcome the challenges of infertility,"* she explained, allaying any unfounded fears they may have about the unusual dynamics of a surrogacy relationship.

Though wonderful, the nine months of pregnancy is always a hormone-induced emotional rollercoaster with a plethora of unexpected twists and turns and surprising dips and loops, and that last month brims with expectation every waking minute, inviting emotional exhaustion by the time the ride ends. The end of the surrogacy introduced a new dimension, because I coveted a bevy of hopes and dreams and fears not just for the baby, but for the intended parents as well. I cried myself to sleep several nights in those final few weeks. Not because I suffered from sadness. Not because I felt confused. Not because I harbored any regrets. But because on top of being exhausted, the hope I carried for this baby totally overwhelmed me. I knew I carried all of the dreams of her family-to-be as well, and I fervently wished for a perfect delivery, a perfect baby.

I worried in the dark space of the night before I could finally fall gently asleep on my pillow: *Have I done everything I can to make this come out right? Will it?* Crying served as a natural release of the worries and pressures that built up inside me over the course of the waking day, so I could sleep peacefully, ready to embrace the next day with a light heart. Afraid that Robert would worry that I had finally started to crumble under the weight of the surrogacy, I waited to let loose my tears until he fell asleep to avoid scaring him unnecessarily. Better to keep it to myself, I thought.

In those last few weeks, in the midst of the heartfelt calls and notes of support from far-flung friends and family touched by the surrogacy, I received a card from Henry's father, a grandfather-to-be, and formerly my Uncle Hank. Henry's parents had divorced early on and I because I was related to Henry through our mothers, I had not seen Hank more than a handful of times over the last thirty years. When I opened the mailbox that afternoon and pulled out an envelope with his name neatly printed on the return address, I smiled with surprise and curiosity. While I had fleetingly considered his response to the surrogacy in the beginning, in truth, because we maintained no direct contact with each other, I had quickly forgotten about his perspective on our venture.

I opened the card to his meticulous block printing style, and sensed the thoughtful care and effort infused into his chosen words of thanks. He wrote, in part, "*I CAN NOT IMAGINE ANYONE GIVING A GREATER GIFT THAN THE GIFT OF LIFE. A GIFT TO HENRY, LAUREN AND THE CHILD,*" signed by *A GRATEFUL GRANDFATHER TO BE.* Our surrogacy, his heartening note reminded me, had become a journey that touched many lives, and, I like to imagine, brought all our lives closer together, like the piecing together of a quilt, sewn with delicate threads that bonded us to each other. While the threads that linked me to Hank remained tenuous, those that bonded him to Henry and Lauren would be strengthened with the joyful celebration of the birth of a granddaughter.

Down to the final two weeks now, Lauren joined me at Dr. Gerber's office for a quick check on May 2nd, and then a final visit on Thursday, May 10th, four days before the scheduled birth. We had made it to the end!

Though a connection to my cousin Henry is what had inspired this journey, Lauren and I had become the partners in pregnancy; one mother living vicariously through another who acted in her place as best she could to be her body, a haven for her baby. We had bonded with each other in admiration and understanding, and while I knew it had not been an easy journey for her, watching someone else carry her child, I think she found that it had not turned out to be as difficult for her as she thought it would be.

Dr. Gerber reviewed with us the 6:00 am hospital check-in on Monday the 14th to be prepped for the scheduled c-section, and outlined again the steps of the delivery plan. We listened and nodded our heads in understanding and silent assent, while she monitored the baby's heart rate and my blood pressure to ensure neither of us labored under any undue stress.

Failing to detect any signs of labor or imminent delivery, Dr. Gerber gave me the go-ahead I requested to attend the wedding of my friend, Stacey, that weekend in Malibu to celebrate with old friends, two hours from Scripps Hospital in Encinitas. She cautioned me, though, to be aware of any significant changes in my physical well-being before then, and to be aware of the possibility that I could be compelled to deliver the baby at an unknown hospital in Los Angeles if labor started and progressed before we could make it back to San Diego.

Lauren generously assured me that she and Henry were comfortable with Dr. Gerber's permission, not wishing to deprive me of an eagerly anticipated visit with old friends after all I had been through for them with the surrogacy. My prior experience made me acutely aware, however, about the very real and risky possibility of an early labor and delivery, and so I promised myself to honor their permission with my own cautiousness and vigilance, ready and willing to give up on the wedding if there were any indication of an early delivery, hoping desperately the baby would not decide to arrive before Monday.

"Well, it looks like we are all ready for delivery on Monday morning!" Dr. Gerber pronounced proudly as we rose to leave the examination room.

*"Who's **WE**, white man?"* I thought, my father-in-law's often quoted words of Tonto to the Lone Ranger echoing in my head. Dr. Gerber of course would be assisting, and Henry and Lauren, after more than a year of anxious hoping, would be there waiting to welcome their daughter to begin life as a family. But, if I remembered correctly, **I** remained the one who would actually be giving birth, the one who had to prepare to go under the knife; with just a few days to go, the reality of delivery and recovery hit me, the memory of the undesirable pain and difficulty of that experience. And **I** carried the weight of the responsibility inside of delivering a perfect baby to my cousin. Ah, yes, details.

After that final pre-delivery doctor visit, Lauren and I hugged each other goodbye tenderly in anticipation of the birth, both of us speechless at having finally arrived at the moment when everything we had hoped, prepared and dreamed for would actually take place in real time, in just few short days. We had nearly prevailed. We lingered for a few minutes with small talk, looking to reassure, support and validate each other, and though excited, we felt puzzled in a way that our journey would be ending, that the relationship we had created to navigate a surrogate pregnancy would inevitably change now.

We would connect again over the weekend before the big delivery day, when Robert and I made a brief visit to Henry and Lauren's home in Manhattan Beach before Stacey's wedding. I coveted the promise of freedom of that weekend away with Robert to escape to our own little world, luxuriating in some time and space alone to reflect and gather strength and perspective for the big day.

Though certainly physically ready at full-term and admittedly desperate to find myself back inside a less awkward body, I felt I needed every minute of the next ninety hours or so to prepare myself mentally for the birth of the child swimming around inside me. Suddenly it all seemed to be moving so fast, the thousands of steps of the surrogacy steeplechase ending abruptly at the finish line. I had arrived, as with any rewarding endeavor, with reluctance and mixed emotions about it coming to an end, returning to the routine and normal, struggling against the excitement and anticipation of the pivotal conclusion. I knew I would be ready to go, to let go when it came time on Monday morning, but I looked forward to the indulgence of the next few days to wonder and reflect on the path of our journey.

friday, may 11th 2001

THE BiRTH

Hope Arrives

STEPPING BACK DOWN THE STAIRS after my visit to the baby's room at Henry and Lauren's, I slid into the guest room shower, soaking my pregnant body beneath a soothing stream of warm running water, while inside me the baby lay suspended in her own protective liquid shield, oblivious to her destiny to exit my womb and enter the world in thirty-six hours.

I let my eyes close while I leaned my burdensome weight against the slick tile of the shower wall, and imagined the room upstairs alive with the baby's presence, the scent of her newness permeating the space.

Oh my god, this was it.

My joyful and anxious tears spilled into the wetness streaming from the shower head as I contemplated our arrival at the end of an exhausting and magical voyage through surrogacy.

A few minutes later I stepped out onto the bathmat, catching a glimpse of my fertile belly in the vanity mirror as I reached for my towel. I pictured the baby inside me at that moment: ten tiny toes, puckered pink lips, fistfuls of fingers, soft downy skin. Pressing the freshly laundered towel up to my face, I breathed in deeply to quiet my jostling emotions, before drying off and slipping into a gauzy sky blue maternity dress I had purchased for the occasion of Stacey's wedding that evening. I attacked my hair with a brush and blow drier, in an attempt to shape my appearance into a sophisticated image for the night's festivities, and evaluating the final effect in the mirror, I ignored my alarmingly protruding midsection, and stepped out into the foyer confident with my appearance.

My cousin, Wende, and Aunt Pam walked through the front door at that moment, returning from a stroll down to the beach for a breath of fresh air. They had arrived on a plane that morning into LAX to stay with Henry and Lauren for the weekend in preparation for the birth of the baby.

"You're here! You look beautiful, but wait, I have the perfect thing for you," my Aunt exclaimed excitedly when she spied me.

Running over to pick up her purse, she carefully retrieved a small beribboned present from inside its fold and eagerly pressed it in my hand, insisting I open it immediately. Inside, a black velvet jewelry box revealed a sparkling pair of diamond earrings, her gift to me in appreciation of the quest I had chosen to embark upon, transforming her son to a father and making possible the delivery of her granddaughter. As I inserted the brilliant stones into my pierced ears, she beamed with pleasure at her success in finding a way to thank me for my life-changing gift, and I paused to reflect on the complexity of a family surrogacy that could have been difficult with so many people to consider, but had in fact only served to widen the circle of joy.

"I promise we'll call immediately if anything happens," Robert assured Henry and Lauren, as he hurried me out to the door to make it to the wedding on time.

We all hugged, bidding farewell until Mother's Day Brunch the next morning in San Diego. A jittery excitement buzzed through all of us with the baby's arrival now so close; we could feel it coming. Lauren and Henry, giddy with anticipation, followed us out the door and snapped a quick picture of me with Robert, his hand covering my belly bursting with their child. Inside I felt like a dizzy teen-age girl waiting in flustered expectation for that first date with a guy I had crushed on for months, smiling at anything and everything, ecstatic to finally be approaching the pivotal moment, coveting the unfolding of events.

"See you guys tomorrow in San Diego," Henry said with a smile, as he and Lauren turned to go back inside.

Robert quietly accompanied me to the car, concerned about the possibility of the pregnancy shifting portentously that evening, two nights before our scheduled rendezvous at Scripps Memorial Hospital in Encinitas for the delivery. And I walked to the curb quietly too, my own thoughts still lingering on that visit to the baby room upstairs, while at the same time eagerly anticipating a reunion with old friends at the wedding; streams of consciousness drifting in two disparate, but not entirely dissimilar directions. Both a wedding and the arrival of a baby were joyous events that represented new beginnings into unchartered territory, a joining together in life-long commitment, supported by the love of family and friends. For me, the birth of the baby inside of me would end my journey as a surrogate mother, and I wondered, what would be *my* new beginning?

With the shine of my new earrings mirrored by the glow of pregnancy lighting me up from within (finally!), we traveled the short ride up the coast to Stacey's wedding at her brother's Malibu beach house. After I had agonized for the last month about the questionable likelihood of my ability to attend the wedding due to my advanced pregnant state, I arrived exhilarated at the rare opportunity to share an enchanted evening with old friends and stepped out of our car into the magical spring night.

"Keep it close and pointed South," Robert entreated the valet, slipping a bill into his hand and hinting with a not-so-subtle nod to my protruding belly that the need may arise for us to depart the wedding quickly in our get-away-and-get-there-fast car.

Holding my hand, Robert led the way down the winding garden path alive with blooming flowers and into the house abuzz with activity and alight with the warm glow of a myriad candles. We delightedly greeted many friends, chatting animatedly as they caressed my belly admiringly, while we waited for the wedding ceremony to begin in a lovely seaside setting outside framed by the softly sculpted sand dunes of the surrounding beach.

"Pam, there you are. You look great, how are you doing?" my friends asked, one after another.

"I feel really good," I reassured them.

Excited for me, but concerned about my emotional state in these last couple of days before the birth, my college buddies rallied around me with a generous dose of comfort and support, paying tribute at the end of my successful surrogacy journey in the midst of the wedding celebration. I treasured the intimate curtain of friendship that gathered all of us in protectively that magical evening while the bride and groom shared their vows, joining together as a couple amidst that crowd of well-wishers, many of whom I counted as my closest friends.

Following the bride and groom's walk back down the aisle together, I spied my dear friend, Shelli (who had delivered the fateful bloody hormone shot for me months ago) in the back, peacefully cradling a newborn in her arms.

"He's adorable, Shelli," I congratulated her delightedly, kissing her new little one gingerly on top of his head. Gazing at his tender face, unchecked tears clouded my vision as I imagined the baby girl inside me finally on the outside, cradled in the arms of her loving parents too. It would just be a matter of hours.

The band cued up under the tent set up next to the patio for the wedding reception, and between snatches of conversation at a table of college friends, Robert and I squeezed in a few energetic dances under the watchful gaze of the bride's mother. She worried distractedly that with any more physical activity I would be required to leave the reception in the back of an ambulance headed for the local maternity ward. I failed to inform her or anyone else when I did, in fact, experience a contraction shortly after my dancing debut. Not strong enough to double me over or send my to my knees, the contraction proved minor and I breathed through it calmly, choosing to ignore it temporarily so that I could enjoy some more precious time with old friends, albeit returning to the dance floor with a little more restraint. *Hold on baby, not yet*, I pleaded under my breath, knowing she dictated her own timetable.

When the hands on Robert's watch pointed to midnight on that lovely evening, he gently dragged me away amidst a barrage of wishes to make the long late-night drive back to San Diego. Though utterly exhausted after the day's events, another contraction on the first half of our car ride kept me up with anticipation, but wishing to avoid scaring Robert unnecessarily, I kept that piece of intelligence to myself, and thankfully we arrived home around two in the morning without any further signs of labor. Pleased with himself for keeping his end of the bargain to get me back to San Diego with a baby still in my belly, Robert climbed into bed next to me and we both passed out immediately.

The next morning arrived quickly: Mother's Day Sunday. As I dragged myself out of bed after Robert gently woke me, the house stirred with the frenzied action of eight people showering; my Mom, Dad and niece Casey had arrived two days earlier to be with the kids while Robert and I spent the weekend in Los Angeles and while I stayed in the hospital for the delivery. Dressing and primping for Mother's Day brunch at the Aviara Resort in Carlsbad, half-dressed family members collided into each other in the narrow hallways of our house, while a pot of coffee gurgled on the kitchen counter, the aroma cutting through the morning fog to awaken our sleepy spirits.

Amidst the cries of *where is my shirt?* And *where can I find the iron?* I watched Kellie pause to diligently change the bright yellow plastic number on the refrigerator from "2" to "1"; our countdown of the last month of pregnancy. Only one more day until the baby arrived!

Slowly we gathered up enough momentum to herd everyone out the front door, the eight of us piling good-naturedly into the *big blue bus* after a few misguided attempts at a viable seating arrangement, my less than agile body secure in the roomy co-pilot chair.

We caused a stir when we arrived at the Aviara Resort, spilling out in all directions like a tumbling basket of upended cherry tomatoes, straightening up into a mostly presentable bunch of celery stalks before we walked in the doors of the dining room for brunch. Henry and Lauren greeted us delightedly along with Aunt Pam and Wende, Joyce and Jerry, Lauren's brother, Mark, and his wife, Nicole. Sixteen of us sat down together for an extended Mother's Day celebration, three generations amidst three families of grandparents, mothers, spouses, cousins, siblings and friends, all brought together in excited anticipation of the birth of the miracle surrogate baby inside me.

"Everyone made it! I'm so glad you're all here," Joyce welcomed us joyfully.

"Congratulations on the baby-to-be," the waiter remarked as I sat down. Lauren and I smiled at each other conspiratorially, and I simply nodded graciously, deciding not to divulge the secret truths of our family gathering that morning.

The brunch played out like the passing of a baton, my leg of the relay almost complete and the attention shifting from my nine-month pregnancy to the day of the birth. As we piled our plates high with steaming brunch delicacies, laughed together at family jokes, and unwrapped flowery Mother's Day gifts, I observed with a mixture of pride and thankfulness the three families gathered around that table, all joined together to honor our team effort through surrogacy and Lauren and Henry's impending leap of faith into the realm of parenthood. It did not seem to matter much anymore who carried the baby, who started the race, as the awkwardness of the beginning of our journey had given way to the full-fledged embrace of her imminent arrival at the finish line. I watched the pleasure in my children's faces as they interacted with a bevy of extended relatives, and unknowingly provided them with a foreshadowing of the joyful family togetherness they eagerly awaited with the birth of the baby. Though weary, I sat there contentedly, proud about the race I had run for the team.

We returned home with our appetites and spirits glowingly satiated, my parents, Aunt Pam and Wende joining in a game of baseball with the kids in the backyard, while I rested inside with a much-needed nap to gather my strength for the birth the following day. Later in the afternoon the bustle of family activity stirred up too much overload for my fragile state of mind, and I discretely begged Dad to come to my rescue. He graciously herded the family visitors out to dinner before Henry and Lauren came over to prepare a quiet dinner for me and Robert and the kids the night before the Big Day.

While Lauren tossed a salad and the kids created cards to welcome their new baby cousin into the world, I sank wearily into the couch cushions, the baby heavy inside my belly the unknowing star of the hour. With the video camera rolling to record the experience for posterity, Henry asked Lise to show him where the baby was hiding. She walked over and patted my belly dutifully.

"Is there anything you want to say to her?" Henry asked Duncan next.

"Yes. You are my cousin and I love you," he pronounced decidedly into the camera lens.

After a dinner of excited chatter about the baby's arrival the next morning, the kids climbed into bed that night brimming with anticipation about their new cousin. I am sure it probably seemed to them like they had been waiting forever for the baby to come out.

"Mommy, will we get to come see the baby at the hospital?" Kellie asked.

"Yes, I promise, either tomorrow or the next day," I assured her.

Because all three of the kids would still be fast asleep when we headed out to the hospital at first light, I hugged each of them close in goodbye and asked them to be good to their grandparents while I was away. I would miss them.

Robert and I settled back into our seats at the dinner table to enjoy a last few minutes of time alone with Henry and Lauren. After we sat down, they presented us with a surprise trip for a week of rest and relaxation in a month's time at the luxurious Princeville Resort, on the lush island of Kauai, to reward us for our life-changing journey through surrogacy.

"We wanted to do something special to thank you guys," Henry said.

"Wow! Thanks so much!" we accepted gratefully.

Robert and I had planned to arrange for some time alone together after the surrogacy ended, and we sincerely appreciated their generous gesture, looking forward delightedly to a week in paradise to reconnect and recharge individually and as a couple. We knew we would certainly need a chance to catch our breath after an eventful year.

"Are we ready?" Robert asked when a weighty quiet settled back over us.

Henry and Lauren appeared nervous and excited, unsure of what to expect during the birth the next morning, while Robert and I wondered curiously about sharing a birth with another couple this time around. Ready or not, though, here she comes! Hugging each other warmly, we bid our good nights until our rendezvous at 6am the next morning at the hospital, where in a few hours time the baby would be born.

"I'm so excited!" Lauren gushed.

"See you guys tomorrow," Henry added casually, carefully masking his gut feelings, though I could see in his eyes the anticipation, fear, and excitement all running around just under the surface. It would be a tough night for him, I thought.

After a year with my life on hold, my role as the surrogate would end, and Lauren's role as a Mom and Henry's as a Dad would just begin. They could finally take back control and ownership of their future, after being forced to wait it out cheering from the sidelines for the last year, unable to quarterback. Though they had coached closely and had a hand in the outcome, the execution and fate of our strategy had been in my hands. Now it would be their turn to get in the game.

Overwhelmed with contradictory emotions about the surrogacy coming to a close and disturbed by some intermittent minor contractions, I slept little that night, waking up around 3am and unable to go back to sleep. I lay in bed with my body propped up on the giant maternity pillow that had become the third wheel in our marriage bed, watching the occasional flutter of movement in my belly, stroking it absentmindedly to soothe the baby and my own anxious hesitations.

I wondered and worried about how each of us would feel within those first few moments of delivery, as I longed for her arrival to be the life-changing, awe-inspiring event that I had envisioned for Henry and Lauren when I had first decided to offer to be their surrogate, and I hoped that I could lie there serenely rejoicing in her arrival when I delivered her to her parents. I wished that in one pivotal moment her perfect little appearance would overwhelmingly surpass the hopes and dreams that we all had cautiously embraced.

Though our long voyage through surrogacy had already altered my perspective on life, I knew that the birth of the baby would be the essential moment when I delivered on my promise, the culmination of all my efforts and desires, and I wondered how that would change me. Would it? And while excited to finally deliver the baby to her parents, I realized that my status and role as surrogate would change abruptly after the birth, and I worried about how I would replace the excitement and exhilaration of surrogacy when I returned to my normal everyday life. Throughout the pregnancy I had wondered if people who found out about the surrogacy would look at me and think me special for agreeing to carry a baby for someone else. I wondered now if, after the birth, people would even remember.

I closed my eyes intermittently in an attempt to allow a peaceful slumber to draw me in, but my heightened state of anticipation would not allow me to relax. In truth, I guarded gingerly those last few solitary hours in the quiet of the night to reflect on the events and emotions of the last year, holding on to some last time alone to commune with the baby inside me, preparing us both for the end of our journey and the commotion of the next day. Like my preparation for a gymnastics meet, I found essential the quiet time to gather my thoughts and focus them on my purpose and the personal meaning of my goal, quieting my mind so that I could enter the arena centered, committed and confident that I could succeed. I prepared myself for the moment the baby would take her first breath outside my body, when our connection would be severed, ending her dependence on me for her life. I knew the time had come for her to exit my insulated womb, and I was not afraid or hesitant about giving her back to Henry and Lauren, but because, unlike with my own children, her physical presence in my life would end abruptly with her arrival, I cherished those last hours cradling closely our intimate connection.

Robert and I snuck out the door quietly in the wee hours of the morning, our hospital bags packed with snacks, cameras, clothes and magazines, speeding the six minutes down the empty freeway to Scripps Hospital and arriving ten minutes early. Hurry up and wait.

We pulled our car into the parking lot and waited for Henry and Lauren to arrive and for the front doors of the hospital to open. While we sat there in the quiet confines of the car, simultaneously exhausted and exhilarated, a last minute fear suppressed successfully until that moment crept into my semi-conscious brain, and I turned to Robert suddenly.

"What if the baby isn't o.k.?" I questioned agitatedly.

I worried about failing everyone when the stakes were so strato-spherically high, and I couldn't even begin to imagine how I would be able to continue, to even look Henry and Lauren in the eyes, if that happened. Robert held my fearful eyes in his reassuring gaze and pro-nounced confidently his unquestioned opinion.

"She will be perfect," he decreed. I knew I loved that guy. At that moment he said exactly what I needed to hear when I desperately need-ed it most.

Henry and Lauren drove up within a few minutes and we greeted each other good morning with a wave and anxious smiles. Awkwardly exiting our cars with a sense of restrained urgency, like runners at the starting line of a crowded race charged with forward momentum in anticipation of the gun, we strode quickly over to begin our adventure inside those hospital doors with the adrenaline pumping furiously in-side our thinly masked exteriors.

We hugged quickly inside the lobby before hurrying down to the hospital labor room where I slid into my standard issue hospital gown, requisite open back laced with multiple ties, and scooted into the bed to be hooked up to the monitors. The baby's heartbeat echoed in the room, while Robert studied the markings on the paper spewing out of the machine registering my uterine activity. Though I could barely feel them, to our surprise significant contractions had begun in earnest again, right on cue for delivery.

"See that. I guess this baby is ready to come out today," Robert said.

Working through our pre-event jitters with a few anxious giggles, we were distracted by the business-like routine as the nurses prepped me for surgery and proceeded with the paperwork for all of us to sign (including our reiterated request for Lauren and Henry to be named as the parents on the birth certificate). The hospital had briefed nurs-es Barbara and Sonya thoroughly on the surrogacy situation and they appeared genuinely excited to be a part of the unique delivery that morning, looking back and forth curiously between us to gauge our emotional state and evaluate the group dynamic.

The quiet of anticipation soon overcame us as we all contemplated the seriousness of the moment. I could feel my whole body begin to tense with anxiety and I could see Robert's concern for me reflected in the tightening of his facial features. Lauren appeared overly bright-eyed with anxious excitement, while Henry moved constantly around the room, keeping busy to calm his nerves; checking the camera, checking his bag of supplies, organizing whatever he could lay his hands on. Just then the nurses handed each of my three birthing partners a surgical suit to pull on over their street clothes to prepare for the O.R., complete with blue gauzy shower hat, mask and booties, presenting a comical picture that resembled a costume call for another Saturday Night Live skit.

"Now that's a good look, you guys," I commented, smiling, the comedy breaking through the building tension just before the nurses wheeled me into the operating room. *Ready.*

The cold metallic surface of the O.R. table aggravated my nascent anxiety, causing me to shake uncontrollably for a few minutes as I sat there hunched over vulnerably, awaiting the poke of the anesthesiologist's epidural needle, acutely aware now of the surgery I would endure before we could celebrate the baby. I froze in pain momentarily as the needle entered my spinal column, wondering for a flash on that table what I had been thinking when I had offered to be a surrogate, to submit myself to a surgical invasion.

Finally, the anesthesia took charge of my involuntary muscle control and numbed my lower body into a more comfortable paralyzed sleep. As I lay down on the operating table, Dr. Gerber and her partner, Dr. Hoppe, entered the room prepped for surgery, greeting me quickly while, all-business, they focused immediately on the surgery purpose, protocol and procedure. Robert, Henry and Lauren surrounded me protectively at the head of the operating table.

"Your strong stomach muscles are getting in the way!" Dr. Gerber complained jokingly as she cut into me with a surgical knife, lightening for a moment the mood in the room as we all held our breath waiting for the baby to emerge. Her attempt to engage me with brief conversation felt like a lifeline, a caring connection that relieved some of my anxiety while she worked away diligently, so that I felt less like a body up for sacrificial slaughter.

As we waited for the doctors to open me up, I focused on relaxing the tension in the parts of my body not numbed by anesthesia, and looked to Robert by my side for comfort, where he stoically sat with love and concern in his eyes, determined as my support system to avoid passing out in the O.R. Beyond him I could see Henry and Lauren, their encouraging expressions mixed with anxiety, controlled panic, helplessness and uncertainty of the unknown, pleading for our shared desire of an easy, successful conclusion. Though the doctors worked quickly, the silence seemed to last forever.

"Almost there!" Dr. Gerber reassured us, as we waited with baited breath. More silence.

"Well, hi there, sweetheart," she said finally.

I peered anxiously as the doctors lifted her above the sheet tented in front of me so I could see her for myself. Lauren moaned with a soulful release of joy and awe, the baby let out an impassioned cry to announce her arrival, and Henry stared speechless through the lens of his video camera. Catching a glimpse of that perfect little body held aloft by Dr. Gerber, and closely studying Henry and Lauren's response, I realized suddenly that my gift had actually, finally become a reality. Stupefied, I smiled tiredly with elated relief at our success, as I let my head fall back on the pillow.

"She looks beautiful, Pam," Dr. Gerber assured me.

Tears swarmed my eyes, each one straining with the physical and emotional struggle of our journey, the taxing drain of a long road of hope and anticipation, ending here, finally, at our coveted destination.

Relieved to discover that the baby arrived in perfect health, I could let those irrational fears of the unknown be swept away.

Turning to follow Henry and Lauren's expressions of rapture, I watched the pediatrician gently place the baby in the incubator. After months and months of complex preparation, she entered the world so quickly and easily; all seven pounds and nine ounces of her. And while I might be inclined to wax poetic about it all feeling like a dream, in truth every moment in that O.R. imprinted itself on my consciousness in a black and white graphically real fashion, my senses heightened to record objectively every stark detail in that room, unlike the diffused reality of most of my memories. This was as real as it gets.

While Dr. Gerber and Dr. Hoppe worked quickly to sew me back together again, Robert sat with me, both of us overwhelmed by the magnitude of the big picture, the amazing reality of actually delivering a baby for another couple, reaching the climactic conclusion of the last year of our time, energy, thoughts, and commitment devoted to the quest of surrogacy. Robert and I looked at each other speechless in wonder. We had actually done it.

I focused my attention on the tiny life carrying forth in that incubator, connected to her hovering parents by an infant grasp on their pinky fingers, one in each hand. While Henry and Lauren gazed at her speechless, the pediatrician checked her vital signs amidst the beeping monitors, attending to her immediate post-birth needs and pronouncing her perfectly healthy. Remarkably calm, Henry cut the umbilical cord through which my body had nourished his daughter for our nine month journey; a bellybutton would form there as the only visible reminder of our connection.

That life which had begun as an embryo frozen in storage for a year, had been thawed and transferred by fertility doctors into my uterus, had been protected carefully for nine months on loan in my belly, and had developed and grown into this miracle of precious life. Baby Hope had arrived.

Swaddled into a blanket burrito, she melted into Henry and Lauren's arms, home at last. They carried her over to me laying there helplessly while the doctors put me back together, to share their joy of her arrival with me.

"Here she is, Pam. You did it," Henry admired. She looked beautiful to me.

After placing her back in the incubator, Henry and Lauren followed Hope out of the operating room when the pediatric nurse wheeled her away, and Robert stayed while the doctors worked to finish sewing me up. The joy of a shared birth gave way to the lonely starkness of surgery in that operating room. I felt tired and disconnected, out of sorts and in pain, the anesthesia failing to mask my discomfort from the doctors tugging and pulling at the several layers of my insides. My purpose had ended, my belly empty now, torn apart, I lay there partially numb in both body and spirit. Dr. Gerber, sensing my disorientation and disillusion, leaned over to encourage me.

"Congratulations, Pam, she's perfect," she applauded. Her comment served to snap me back away from the precipice to focus on the miracle of my accomplishment.

"Look at me and breathe," Robert gently commanded, squeezing my hand tightly.

Finally, the nurses wheeled me back into recovery, a roomy, private post-partum room with two beds and a window out onto the courtyard. Henry and Lauren left baby Hope to give me some privacy while the nurses worked diligently to make me comfortable, covering me with blankets, checking my vital signs, etc.

Within a few minutes I unexpectedly started shaking uncontrollably, and Nurse Barbara quickly scooped up Hope from her bassinette and laid her on my naked chest in an effort to calm me. I relaxed into her warmth immediately, the shaking that racked my body subdued by her touch, a craving for contact since the doctors removed her from my belly finally satisfied. Robert marveled at my body's automatic response to her presence and the nurse's intuitive understanding of my primal need to hold Hope in my arms, before my body could let her go.

"I just thought you might need to have a chance to hold her," Barbara whispered sympathetically.

Caressing Hope gently, I could finally take a deep breath in relief. "We did it," I whispered to her. "Oh my God, we did it. Thank you," I said, as the tears welled up in my eyes once again in relief.

Henry and Lauren returned to our recovery room to sponge bathe Hope and change her first diaper after I had recovered. As Hope warmed up in the incubator, Lauren rubbed her tiny toes and exclaimed sympathetically, "She's cold!"

"Well, what do you expect? She was in a freezer for a year!" Henry responded mischievously. Giddy with success, the months of anxious anticipation at an end, Lauren giggled along with me at Henry's light-hearted attempt at infertility humor.

I watched Henry enraptured with Hope as he cautiously wrapped her up in soft flannel baby blankets and held her blissfully in his arms, rocking her back and forth in an intimate mutual connection, without any care beyond the immediate world of his infant daughter. I felt honored to be allowed to witness their bonding.

"Pam, she is perfect," Lauren declared with appreciative awe. I had done my job and I could take enormous pride in that now.

After a few hours holding her in their arms and gazing rapturously at her innocent beauty, Henry and Lauren invited Robert out to breakfast for some much needed solid nourishment. Lauren first brought Hope over to my bed and placed her tenderly in the curve of my arms, thanking me for the amazing miracle of her arrival. Lauren emanated a calmness now, at peace with a beautiful baby to hold to trump the challenges of the previous year of cancer and infertility, no longer at the whim of events outside of her control.

Alone with Hope after they left, an intimate moment to share just between the two of us outside of my womb, I marveled at her sweet face, caressed her soft skin and breathed in her heavenly smell. Whispering again my thanks to her for the chance to share in her arrival, I celebrated our connection to each other in that quiet, empty space; though undeniably unlike the mother-child connection I felt at the birth of my own babies, her presence touched and comforted me.

Lauren and Henry invited their families to come visit in the early afternoon, but before they arrived at the hospital I started shaking uncontrollably again with the pain and emotion of my experience that morning, my body trembling with the instinctive need to hold the newborn I had birthed. Nurse Barbara quickly brought Hope over to me again and laid her on my chest, my body relaxing immediately into the magnetic connection between us, the shakes dissipating quickly, while Henry and Lauren watched wide-eyed and Robert marveled again at her primal power to soothe my panic into retreat.

Though my body's uncontrollable crying out and Hope's power to calm me initially may have scared Henry and Lauren, perhaps fueling a momentary fear about the nature and depth of our connection, I gave them words of reassurance to help them understand that I was not emotionally conflicted about letting her go, my body simply needed time to let go physically.

I recovered in short time and in the late afternoon the anxious grandparents arrived to finally meet their granddaughter. Aunt Pam came through the hospital room door first, a delighted smile lighting her face as she laid her eyes on Hope. Happy to be a grandmother, and thankful that Henry had become a father, she rocked Hope back and forth in her arms serenely. Joyce arrived moments later, immediately transfixed by the presence of her granddaughter; overcome with the emotion of the moment, her eyes widened in wonder as she gazed at Hope.

"I am speechless. For the first time in my life, I am speechless," Joyce said simply. Jerry, moved by the sight of his wife holding Lauren's baby daughter, remained speechless in communion next to her.

"You have a beautiful granddaughter," I pronounced to all the grandparents.

"Thanks to you," my aunt answered, loving gratitude in her eyes.

Wende stood in awe of the delicate beauty of her new niece and her brother's transformation into his role as a father, while Mark and Nicole seemed both astounded and afraid of their niece's precious fragility. The family's expressions of thanks and their enraptured interactions with baby Hope fed my soul and spirit, as I observed many unshed tears of joy and relief hanging in the balance that afternoon.

Before the relatives left reluctantly that evening, each one of them inquired touchingly about my physical and emotional well-being, and made a point of thanking me tenderly, fervently for bringing them this little miracle. When Jerry approached to thank me, I sensed his concern for my health while he discretely evaluated my current condition with the keen and practiced eye of an expert physician. Aware of the medical strain and discomfort of cesarean surgery mixed in with the emotional upheaval of a surrogate birth and the attending commotion, he appeared sensitive to the toll they had taken on my body and my state of mind. Though he refrained from mentioning it directly to me, I appreciated his concern for my compromised condition.

With a precious few quiet moments to myself that evening after everyone else headed out to dinner, I gathered my strength to chance a trip over to the bathroom on my own. Cautiously sliding my legs gently over the side of the bed, I leaned my weight on my elbow and pushed up to a seated position, dangling my feet over the edge of the bed. I let out a tense breath between gritted teeth, willing the pain in my abdomen to remain at bay, while my bare feet touched the cold linoleum floor as I shifted my weight onto weakened legs. I paused to peer out through the open blinds into the courtyard outside, where the lack of movement mirrored the suspension of time shut inside that room, disengaged from the pattern of daily life and world events continuing in motion beyond.

Stooping over at the waist like a struggling old lady, hospital gown flapping subtly open in all the wrong places, I shuffled my way around the corner of the bed, employing the IV pole attached to me as a crutch for my walk to the other side of the room. Inadvertently banging the pole up against the bathroom door, I nudged my way awkwardly inside, scooting around the side of the sink and closing the door heavily behind me. As I lowered my weight onto the abrupt coolness of the smooth toilet seat underneath me, I dropped my head between my knees and exhaled in exasperated relief. So much effort for such a trivial mission; in comparison space travel seemed a snap, for at least astronauts can rely on the assistance of mission control. Resting there helplessly, I heard voices drifting back into the hospital room, and I felt eternally thankful for the weight of the door between me and that room full of expectations.

Overwhelmed by the events of the day and the climactic conclusion of the expectations of the last year, I let go then, releasing a silent flood of unchecked tears down my cheeks.

What had I been thinking to believe I possessed the courage and strength to carry off a surrogate pregnancy? I felt helplessly weak and the pain of moving around proved to be almost unbearable. I observed my reflection in the mirror over the sink, and felt oddly disconnected from the haggard face staring back at me, drained of life and crowned by a limp tangle of hair. I splashed some water over my eyes, rubbing in the cool wetness vigorously, in an attempt to wipe away the layers of weariness and rediscover my old self underneath.

Leaning on the sink, head in my hands, I contemplated the impossibility of reversing time back to the pivotal moment when I had offered to sacrifice myself up to be a surrogate. Reversing time and erasing all of it: the offer, the scores of pain-in-the-ass (literally) hormone shots, the months of day after day nausea, the lack of energy, the c-section, and finally the damned inability to even take a pee without losing control of myself.

Forcing myself to stand up straight, I gulped down a few deep breaths to try to regain my composure, knowing that on the other side of that door Henry and Lauren awaited me, anxious to reassure themselves that I remained in good spirits, sympathetic to the pain of my recovery. I summed up the strength to wipe away my tears and emerged from that sanctuary to shuffle back to my bed with a forced smile.

Just then a nurse swept in with a bouquet of beautiful flowers for me from my friend, Shelli. A note attached said simply, *"You did a really great thing! We love you."* Smiling genuinely at her encouraging words, I remembered to focus on why I had chosen to be there and what I had accomplished, instead of the pain and frustration of the moment. *I did a really great thing.* I had momentarily lost control, but the moment of regret quickly dissipated as I looked over at my cousin enthralled with his new baby daughter, and repeated those few words from Shelli as a soothing mantra in my head. *I did a really great thing. I did a really great thing.*

My Dad and niece, Casey, arrived later that night to visit, each of them holding Hope cautiously and rewarding me with gentle hugs of support that nourished me. Robert came to stay with me later, bringing with him a note from Duncan generated in big block colorful letters on the computer at school that morning.

"HI MOM! I LOVE YOU......I HOPE YOU HAVE THE BABY ......LOVE DUNCAN" it said. I smiled through tears at the simple words of love and encouragement from my son that somehow managed to make everything o.k.

At my bedside, Robert appeared tired and somewhat frazzled from his multiple roles that day; he had the unenviable position of juggling the responsibilities of a hospitalized wife, visiting in-laws, young children at home, as well as a hectic work schedule. Later that night alone in bed thinking about the toll of the day's events and the underlying chaos of the past year, he called to tell me that despite his concerns for my health and the post-surgery reality, bottom line he mostly just felt really proud of us.

"I have no regrets," he said.

"Me either," I agreed, before hanging up.

Lauren and I whispered to each other across the room while Hope slept in the bassinette that night.

"She's beautiful, Lauren. I can't believe she's actually here," I said.

"She's a little miracle," Lauren agreed, before we both finally fell asleep in our hospital beds.

I smiled contentedly when Hope's cries awakened me later in the night, only too happy to abandon my sleeping dreams to the precious reality of the successful conclusion of our surrogacy venture. Lauren tried to quiet Hope by rocking her, without success, but conscious that Hope's protection and well-being now resided solely in the care of Lauren and Henry, I waited awhile before interfering. Most new mothers do not have to share a hospital room with a woman who carried their child, and I tried to tread lightly so as not to overstep, because she deserved the privilege to figure things out on her own.

"You might want to try feeding her, she could be hungry," I eventually suggested delicately, prompted by the sensation of nature's milk coursing through my awakening breasts. Lauren, relieved to be given a solution, quieted Hope with a bottle of formula to satisfy her.

In the morning I pumped my full breasts to retrieve the *liquid gold* colostrum for Henry and Lauren to feed their baby, promising them to continue pumping for at least a few days so Hope could benefit from the precious antibodies present in the first few days of breast milk. While recognizing the inappropriateness of breastfeeding someone else's baby, regardless of whether I had carried her inside me, and without any desire to do so, I still wanted to deliver to Hope the milk that nature provided to protect her entrance into the big wide world.

That morning the nurses removed my I.V. and catheter, and with the freedom to move around more easily and the medication working effectively to reduce my pain, the day began much more comfortably, and the overwhelming feelings of the night before had disappeared. Though I moved slowly, easing myself into different positions on the hospital bed and shuffling back and forth to the bathroom, I found no need to hurry and instead took advantage of the opportunity to literally rest on my accomplishments. I treasured this time to relax and enjoy the moment, wrapping it around me and snuggling deep inside it, pulling it up over me like the sheets on my hospital bed and screaming to myself in a whisper, *Oh my God, I did it!*

Dad and Casey returned that morning on their way down to the airport to say a brief goodbye. Dad approached my bed tentatively with tears in his eyes and struggled to whisper something to me.

"I am so proud of you, sweetheart."

"Thanks, Dad," I said, touched by his sincerity, hugging him close.

"I stayed up all night kicking myself for not saying that to you yesterday. Robert suggested I stop by on my way out this morning to tell you how I felt," he said.

My father is probably better than most men of his generation at sharing his feelings, but there are times when he has trouble communicating his emotions with words that escape him in intimate moments. I am lucky my husband enjoys an open and mutually respectful relationship with my dad, and he had wisely validated Dad's feelings, encouraging him to share how he felt with me. Surrogacy can be awkward, and while for the most part everyone in the family had embraced it, they were still unsure at times about the appropriate code of conduct. In that case I think it is always best to just go with what is in your heart, and that is exactly what Robert had encouraged my Dad to do.

Robert brought Lise by later that morning before he took her to preschool because she had asked for me repeatedly, but I could tell when she came in by the unsure look on her face that the unfamiliarity of me in that hospital room overshadowed her excitement to see me and the baby. Still just 3 ½ years old, she had probably envisioned the baby simply popping out and expected her invincible mommy to be back up immediately and running around as usual.

Staring at me, confused and uncertain, she confessed to Robert in whispers that my messed up hair looked funny. My obvious infirmity scared my compassionate little girl, so I tried my best to reassure her. Comforting her with the ritual motherly duty of brushing her hair and putting it up in clips, I hugged her closely before she left for school.

I looked in the mirror after they left and no wonder I scared her; I looked like a mess. My own unkempt hair stuck out in a fuzzy rats nest from lying in bed all day and night, and the harsh hospital light magnified my pale, post-surgery face, no makeup or brush having touched me for 24 hours, resulting in a pasty witch look that I resolved to do my best to remedy before the rest of the visitors arrived that day.

Karen Chernekoff, our surrogacy psychologist, was the first to visit later that morning to congratulate all of us and check in with the hospital staff to ensure the accommodations for our surrogacy birth had proceeded smoothly and appropriately.

"How are you feeling, Pam," Karen asked genuinely when we shared a private moment, focusing her undivided attention on me as she sat down next to my hospital bed.

"I'm great. I feel better today, just tired." I responded. And I meant it; the overwhelming excitement of the previous day mellowing now to enjoyment and appreciation.

After inquiring more directly into my state of mind and assuring herself of my healthy response to the birth events, Karen left my bedside encouraged by my attitude. With words of approval and support, she had presented me with a tube of scented lotion to soothe my weary body and a card to honor my journey as a surrogate mother. She had helped us be better prepared for the surrogacy and the birth, smoothing out any potential bumps in the road before they had appeared on the horizon; I fully appreciated now the structure provided by psychological and legal counsel to facilitate a beautiful journey through an awkward and unknown landscape.

When Karen left the hospital after admiring Hope and speaking with Henry and Lauren, I slid the card from her out of its envelope. *"You've changed the world and made a miracle! I hope......that you treasure this experience as one of your life's highlights and a reminder of your incredible generosity....."*, she wrote. I have always considered it one of my shortcomings, actually, that I am not naturally given to generosity on a day-to-day basis; but I thought, maybe she was right. I could point to this journey now, embarked upon with a selfless act of love and a wish to make a difference, as proof of my generous spirit. And I would always treasure the surrogacy as a highlight of my life's experience, with Hope's birth and delivery to her parents captivating the essence of a miracle for me.

The family visitors arrived again later that morning, and the room swirled with activity; while the day before all had been fairly quiet in relief, reverence and contentment at the surrogate delivery of a newborn baby, today in contrast began with celebration and excitement.

Joyce brought flowers for me and chocolate cake from the Aviara that they had presented her in commemoration of becoming a grandmother. And I found tickets for our family to see the Lion King theatrical production in Los Angeles tucked inside a card she handed me that said, *"For your extraordinary gift of love, we are so grateful. Thank you just doesn't seem enough."* But the best gift Joyce brought with her that morning proved to be words she confessed in relief to Lauren, relief that had flooded her the day before when she had held Hope in her arms.

"That was the first good night of sleep I have had in the two years since you were diagnosed with cancer," Joyce confessed in an emotional whisper.

Those words caught my breath and stung my eyes with tears. Looking from Joyce's perspective as a mother with a fierce instinct to protect her child from harm, I could understand her fear and suffering, and I treasured my role in giving her finally some peace of mind. Out of the long, anxious passage from the scare of death emerged the promise and joy of new life: baby Hope.

When Aunt Pam and Wende visited our hospital room that morning to hold Hope one more time before they flew out of town, my aunt wrapped me in a big warm hug, emotion brimming in her eyes, thanking me repeatedly for giving Henry a little girl. I knew in my heart that she took great comfort in my connection to Henry, in the boundless nature of family ties that ran deep and true enough to have inspired me to give to him so generously. A quiet and deep gratitude permeated the blanket of joy enveloping our room that day, a gratitude I found infinitely rewarding as I proudly observed thankful family become enamored with Hope.

Our venture had touched many lives, and the commotion and emotion surrounding this birth were unprecedented in my experience. I received calls from a wide cast of friends and family members with congratulations and wishes for a quick recovery, as well as words of admiration for my accomplishment. I took infinite pride in their words and nourishment from the flurry of attention, the likes of which I had not experienced since my wedding day. Surrogacy represented another, different kind of passage to celebrate and add to my life story.

Echoed in the voices of those I loved I could hear some thoughtful words of concern for my current emotional state, but I reassured them that rather than mourning a loss, I found myself rejoicing, my heart fulfilled by virtue of my life-changing gift.

Lauren and Henry left the hospital to eat lunch with family that day, so Robert and I enjoyed some treasured time alone with Hope. We shared then with each other our relief and pride that all of our hopes and efforts had proven exceedingly fruitful, and our appreciation that our combined generosity and mutual support had managed to create a miracle that transformed people's lives deeply and irrevocably. Lying down on the hospital bed next to me with Hope snuggled between us, Robert looked me in the eyes.

"We will always have this," he said, "to look back on and know that we are generous; to draw strength from that."

We gazed from each other back and forth to Hope, wonder and joy mirrored in our eyes. Our faith and belief in each other rooted in a desire to make others happy had initiated a life-affirming experience so deeply moving and powerful that an intimate, wordless magic now hovered around us in an embracing bubble. The bubble would last, we knew, for only a few precious minutes before it popped, its protective enclosure dissipating into the thin air of external reality, but we trusted that the power of the magic we had created within it would touch us forever.

Joyce and Jerry returned late that afternoon with gifts of brightly colored puppets for my children, and loaded down with snacks from a shopping spree at Trader Joe's to share, while they said goodbye, giddily looking forward I sensed to the days, weeks, months and years ahead with their new granddaughter.

Kellie, Duncan and Lise arrived shortly before they left to meet their new cousin. They celebrated the reward of accomplishment we had shared with a party in the hospital, diving into Joyce's chocolate cake, performing a show with their new puppets, and snapping pictures of Hope with the disposable cameras Lauren had given them ahead of time for the occasion. As young children, they were easily distracted by the puppets and cake, but there was no mistake they were enthralled with Hope. Each of them, in turn, wearing surgical masks and having scrubbed their hands clean beforehand per our adamant instructions ("No germs, mommy, see?!"), proudly and gingerly held their baby cousin in their arms in the rocking chair, eyeing her curiously as they marveled at her presence outside my belly. And their eyes continued to turn toward her in the quiet moments between the celebrating.

Later, Robert returned the kids to play at home with their grandmother, and then joined me again back in the hospital room that evening to relax, rest and recuperate in that hushed cocoon, privileged to watch Henry and Lauren and Hope become a family. After enjoying the quiet time together to reflect on the gift we had given each other, Robert and Henry left, and Lauren, Hope and I settled in for another night together. Joyce called just before we fell asleep.

"If there is anything you need, please let me know…….. anything you need EVER," she insisted. The emotion behind those emphatic words made crystal clear for me the dramatic impact my choice to be a surrogate for Lauren left on an eternally grateful grandmother.

Hope woke up a couple of times that night to eat, and I humbly watched Lauren enthralled with her, her every little sound and ounce of being. In thirty-six hours baby Hope had magically, irrefutably captivated those who now loved her unconditionally. I smiled to myself. Everything was as it should be, as I had hoped it would be.

Henry arrived in the morning shortly after we woke up, a box of muffins in his arms, energy and purpose in his step, announcing that he had already serviced the car at the local oil change shop, determined that the ride home with baby Hope to Manhattan Beach would be smooth and uneventful.

Lauren and I exchanged conspiratorial smiles. I had learned a lot about my cousin over the course of the last year, and especially over the last few days in the close confines of our hospital room. Foremost, he is a manic organizer/planner/ preparer; he's the guy you want planning a group summit of Mt. Everest or your 40th birthday party. He had managed to walk miles in our hospital room in our two days there, back and forth, organizing and reorganizing, driven to distraction by disarray, and desperate to perform a productive duty in his role as the protective father. (Hence, the oil change.) That's a guy thing, I think, the doing part.

But I had also seen him enveloped with a sense of calm when he held his baby girl, no longer fidgety to do, but revealing his sweet paternal side, as he stroked his daughter's cheek tenderly, gazing unabashedly at her perfection. Though it is true Hope will learn every minute from her father over the course of her life, he will learn from her even more profoundly about himself and his capacity to love.

While I rested, Henry and Lauren packed up the baby clothes, diapers, gifts and accessories in the room to prepare to finally bring their little girl home later that morning, our journey now coming to an end. As I watched them get ready to leave I felt conflicted, not wanting them to leave me all alone, not ready for the surrogacy to end altogether, yet ready to move beyond the hospital room and knowing it was time for them to start off on their own, to go home and be a family. When my cousin finished packing, he tiptoed over to my bedside, gently nudging me awake, and I opened my eyes to find myself gazing directly at the serene expression of a beautiful sleeping Hope.

"Lauren and I are going to go pack up our clothes at the hotel and grab some breakfast, before we return to check out of the hospital," he whispered, laying hope down gently on the bed in the curve of my arm. Henry and Lauren kissed us both a temporary and reluctant goodbye, and tiptoed out the hospital room door, leaving us there alone for a couple of precious quiet hours together.

Deeply grateful for that deliberately orchestrated opportunity they had so graciously given me alone with Hope, I prepared to say goodbye. Undeniably, a connection coursed through us, established during nine months of pregnancy and transformed through her birth into a lasting link to each other; a bond unlike that between a parent and child, but a visceral connection born out of our unique journey together.

As I curled my body into that precious shape, bundled carefully in a swath of receiving blankets, I took comfort in the miracle of every newborn breath. One hand escaped from the swaddling, curled tightly in an impossibly tiny fist, and grabbed instinctively at my pinky finger, holding my whole body hostage in its fragile grip.

A peaceful warmth flooded me, as silent tears of wonder and joy slipped faintly in fresh, warm drops down my cheeks and onto the newborn nightgown. Gazing down at that baby's sweet innocence, I reflected on my decision to engage in this crazy, inspired adventure called surrogacy. The difficulty, pain and sacrifice exacted by our quest slipped away like a silk sheath, as I shared that time and space together with this new life I had helped bring into the world. It was our moment just to be and I soaked it in contentedly, passing away the hour basking in her perfection.

"Goodbye sweetheart. Thank you. Thank you for choosing me," I said to her.

When my cousin and his wife returned to my hospital bedside, I placed their baby in their loving arms with a mixture of joy and sadness, but without a speck of regret. We had all truly created a miracle together and what an awesome adventure we had shared.

Henry efficiently completed the packing up of Hope's things in the hospital room, while Lauren carefully dressed her in a soft new baby outfit and bundled her safely into her carrier for the ride home to Manhattan Beach.

Robert arrived then with an empty wheelchair he had thoughtfully secured, allowing me the chance to say goodbye to my cousin's new family as they left the hospital. After a few last pictures, he helped me into the chair, steering me down the hall slowly after Lauren and Hope, while Henry ran outside to pull the car up to the curb. We shared celebratory hugs and words of encouragement with the nurses as we made our way through the halls, gliding out through the automatic doors where I had walked in on my own two feet only two days earlier with Hope still kicking inside of me.

The mind boggling jumble of the events and emotions of those days raced through my mind as I sat there quietly in the wheelchair, the finality of the moment hitting me suddenly, robbing me of any words.

Henry had already parked at the front curb, a sense of fatherly purpose in his step as he opened the car doors to pack up his new family. It was noticeably quiet as Lauren held Hope up to me in her carrier, whispering a heartfelt "thank you" in my ear. I kissed each of them goodbye through my tears. Loading Hope carefully into the car and buckling her carrier down in the backseat next to Lauren, Henry closed the doors after them hesitantly, unsure of leaving me there behind; an awkward final moment of separation.

"Goodbye, Pam. I promise we'll call you later," Henry said earnestly as he hugged me, before climbing into the driver's seat. I waved at them through the blurry haze of my tears and the glare of the sunlight bouncing off my glasses, as they drove quietly away from the curb and out of the hospital driveway onto Highway 5 Northbound for home. I tried to yell goodbye after them as the car pulled away, but no sound came out except a muffled grunt. They were gone.

Though heart-wrenching on one level to watch them drive away from me, I proudly watched them begin their rightful journey as a new family. I would miss Hope's presence, but I did not mourn the *loss* of her, for I could not mourn the loss of a baby that I had never claimed as mine.

Society tells us that our natural instinct should be to bond with the baby we carry, and at least one wayward fertility book I came across claims that those instincts make it difficult for a surrogate mother to give up a child that she has carried. Yes, I carried Hope inside me for nine months and experienced the day to day discomfort, exhaustion and joy associated with pregnancy. I never once, though, in the whole time she kicked inside of me, considered her mine. My irrefutable natural instinct told me all along that the baby I carried as a surrogate mother was never mine to *give up*, and it felt like the most natural, joyful act in the world to deliver her *back* to the waiting arms of her parents. I simply provided Hope with a safe place to grow and develop, but her parents truly brought her into this world, acting intently on their wishes and desires. And I had no regrets.

But I did mourn the end of the surrogacy, the loss of the temporary circumstances that had joined me in a precious relationship with Henry and Lauren which had existed suspended outside the course of normal daily events, though the tears I shed then were not of sorrow, but of relief, of overwhelming comprehension at having successfully realized our quest for the miracle of her birth.

We stayed there at the curb for a few minutes frozen temporarily, Robert and I, both of us contemplating their departure, our future, unsure of our next move. Robert found himself left alone with his damaged wife wrapped in a bathrobe, slumped in a wheelchair, drained from the pain of surgery and hormonal emotion of the last couple of days. It took a concerted effort from him not to complain out loud. It just seemed unfair. Nobody, nothing had prepared us for the moment when they drove off with the baby and the excitement and commotion surrounding the surrogacy end abruptly, leaving us to pick up the pieces and fit them back together into a whole again. What happens next?

Struggling to cope with our new circumstances, Robert wheeled me back in the doors of the hospital, both of us numbly quiet, unable to quite grasp that the surrogacy had suddenly ended. Returning to my hospital room, I knew not what to feel, or say, or do, without everyone else there; without the joy of a newborn and new family on which to focus my attention, the color drained from within those walls, and the emptiness of the room sucked the wind out of me. Dazed and unsure, I searched Robert's eyes desperately for answers, and he kneeled down on the floor next to my hospital bed, tears forming as he watched me collapse in confusion, and hugged me close. I cried then, holding on to him, while all those mixed-up emotions and raging hormones coursed through me.

After a few minutes of losing myself, I shook away those feelings temporarily and focused myself back into that empty room; making an effort to look ahead instead of behind, to reach out with a tentative step forward to discover what may come next. Though I worried now that the transition post-surrogacy might not be easy, I comforted myself with the reminder that my loving husband and children patiently waited to help me return to my normal life.

It came time for Robert to get back to work, and hugging me closely goodbye, he reluctantly left me alone in that hospital room to sort through my feelings, while he left to meet his outside obligations. No Hope. No Henry. No Lauren. No husband. In the midst of all that quiet the empty space around me grew expansive and unfamiliar. The phone rang out to displace the quiet a couple of times with congratulations from friends, and then I closed my eyes in hopes of retreating from its melancholy into the safety of a nap.

Just as I drifted off two nurses bustled in, flipping the lights on, noisily snatching the bed curtain closed and switching out the other bed where Lauren had slept for another patient. Though the quiet and empty space around me vanished, the activity outside my curtain failed to fill the emptiness I felt inside. I huddled down under my hospital blankets and focused myself and my thoughts inward. Without Henry and Lauren and Hope, I reasoned objectively, my role as a surrogate over, I had essentially become an ordinary hospital patient taking up space in a hospital bed. Without a baby or the parents to bear witness to our quest, my presence there in the hospital maternity ward, in fact, felt like a farce, c-section scar notwithstanding.

My good friend, Liza, came by to visit me at that moment as the nurses brought the new mother in to take up residence in the bed next to mine. The girl, for that's what she appeared to be, young enough to be in high school, yacked it up with a friend, while her newborn baby slept in the bassinette, and, to my horror, she flipped to *Jerry Springer* on the TV. I could not even begin to fathom why a brand new mother with a beautiful baby to cuddle would turn on the television for mindless, fruitless entertainment; much less choose to turn on the trashiest show out there. What are people thinking?

Liza, appalled at such a sad statement on society, rolled her eyes in disbelief, and I cringed at the actions of my new roommate. Liza tried goodheartedly to distract me from my emotions and the commotion next to me, but when she left a little while later with concern evident on her face and in her voice, she felt damn sorry she could not take me away with her.

I came to the quick realization immediately after she walked out that I could not possibly stand to stay there in that room for a moment longer. Lying there in pain, alone, shoved in a corner, Jerry Springer proved the final insult. I called Robert on his cell phone and begged him to come rescue me. We had anticipated my staying one more night in the hospital to rest from the discomfort of the surgery, but Dr. Gerber had given me the o.k. to leave after 5 pm if I wished, and I could not wait to get the hell out of there.

I needed to have my family around me now, to be surrounded by their love and comforted by their presence. I nearly broke down on the phone with Robert, and while I waited for him to come take me away I covered my ears to halt the ugly attack of those words spewing out of the television on my fragile state of mind. I wanted to pick up that baby and cover her ears too, to protect her for as long as possible from the caustic influence of the outside world.

When Robert arrived and discovered me stashed in the corner of that room, he angrily resolved to get me out of there as quickly as possible. The nurse apologized when he approached her, explaining to him that they had lacked sufficient recovery room space for the new mothers that had delivered that day, and had waited as long as possible to double up on me.

We understood the practical circumstances, but the way they had unceremoniously relegated me to the corner of my room, within a couple of hours of baby Hope leaving, without any initial apology or explanation, had wounded me. They had treated us compassionately and respectfully throughout the rest of my stay, which is what barely kept Robert from laying into them on my behalf, but at that moment I felt like they had tossed me out to sea to end an incredible pilgrimage through surrogacy in a corner by myself, stuck dodging the wave of vitriolic hyperbole from Jerry Springer. We filled out the paperwork to leave the hospital as quickly as possible, and I had never felt so glad to be going home.

The kids welcomed me home with big smiles and gentle hugs when Robert helped me out of the car in our driveway and through the front door. I shuffled down the hall to my bedroom and lay down on my bed carefully, while they covered me with soft blankets and fluffed my pillows, arranging my flowers and cards for me to look at from my sanctuary. Henry and Lauren called shortly afterwards to let me know they had made it home safely and to check in on me, to make sure the transition home from the hospital had gone well and I that I was feeling o.k.

"It was really quiet in the car on the ride home," Lauren said. "I felt really, really bad when we left you at the hospital in a crappy environment with no baby and all of us gone. I didn't feel right," Lauren apologized.

"Don't worry about it, Lauren. I couldn't wait to get out of there, but everything is okay now that I am home, and I am fine," I assured her, before saying good night.

A bright pink card on my nightstand from Kellie shouted lovingly: *"Welcome home mommy. I Love You."*

I relied on the medication to control my pain, and with the kids there to comfort me and Robert and my Mom waiting on me, I breathed with relief, thankful to be home to heal under the protection and care of my family. I smiled appreciatively, ready and at peace with preparing myself to make the transition to life after surrogacy, as far away as possible from Jerry Springer.

THE PARTY'S OVER
Restoration & Reflection

Two nights after arriving back home to recover from the birth, I managed to shuffle to the dining room for Dad's birthday dinner on May 18th, but we retreated to my bedroom for the birthday cake when the post-c-section pain and weariness overcame me, forcing me to lie down.

"Wait, Dad, you can't come in yet!" I stopped him.

I pumped another round of breast milk, while Mom snuck in his new birthday bicycle through the side patio door of the master bedroom. We finally allowed him in with his eyes closed, while the kids joined Robert and Mom in singing happy birthday from my rumpled bed.

Dad's eyes flew open wide like those of a much younger boy when he spied the shiny new bike in the corner of my bedroom, but then closed in disbelief when he spied the bottle of newly pumped breast milk on my nightstand. Shaking his head and laughing simultaneously at the absurdity of the scene, his daughter recuperating in bed from delivering a baby to his nephew, he contemplated this rather unique departure from the birthday celebrations of his past sixty-eight years. At least the bike appeared to be traditional.

That night, instead of birthday cake, I eyed hungrily the square box of See's chocolates resting on my nightstand, my favorite Scotch-mallows® of dark chocolate, chewy caramel and spongy marshmallow centers, a gift from Lauren and Henry on the day I gave birth to Hope. I had not bitten into their savory centers yet, which given my love affair with chocolate could be considered quite a feat in my household, but instead I had left them intact at arms length, savoring the knowledge of their existence while delaying my indulgence, holding on instead to the meaning attached to that gift like I held onto the remnants of the surrogacy.

Though Hope had arrived and I had been released from the hospital days earlier, in truth, for me the surrogacy had failed to end abruptly with those events. Reluctant to let go of the journey that brought Hope into the world, I hesitated to flip the switch and look forward in a new direction that would inevitably leave the surrogacy behind. Content to check in with Henry and Lauren from a distance, without any latent maternal instincts unsuspectingly materializing to cause me to regret her absence, I still found that it would require a conscious effort to step beyond the cocoon of surrogacy. I had traveled on this amazing adventure and when it had finally come to its dizzyingly successful conclusion, I had found it difficult to release myself from its fulfilling hold.

Standing there at the top of the symbolic mountain I had climbed and basking in my accomplishment for a few brief moments, I savored the breathtaking view. Though the birth of Hope represented an individual ending that would shape my world view forever, I realized now I would have to reach out to find the next beginning, the next toehold, the next challenge on my life's pilgrimage.

I reached past the birthday cake that night to open the box of See's, my first bite of chocolate inviting me to step down a path of closure, of transition from surrogate mother back to myself again. Each time

I opened the box of chocolates after the first, I weighed my desire for temporary sweet pleasure against my readiness to take another step toward reality; each deliberate bite of chocolate leading me further down that path as I ate my way slowly through the box, consciously choosing to empty it, allowing the surrogacy to slip bitter-sweetly a bit further from the present into a treasured memory.

I rested in bed recuperating that first week back home, my body propped up for comfort by pillows and my spirits propped up by the comforting acknowledgements I received in the dozens of phone calls, flower deliveries, and visits from friends and family expressing their congratulations and admiration. The flowers marked the passage of time like the box of chocolates, bursting forth colorfully with their cheery fragrant power to heal and restore in those first few days back home, before they slowly began to lose their luster, fading away until Mom recycled them mercifully in the outgoing trash. The cards, though, remained standing on my dresser indefinitely where their words could boldly remind me of the steady love and support that surrounded me.

Henry and Lauren called me every day to inquire concernedly after my health and well being, and to deliver updates on their new little miracle. Our shared attention had shifted from the world inside my belly to Hope's engagement with the outside world, and hearing their joy as parents served to facilitate my transition away from surrogate mom and refocused my attention on the outcome of our quest.

And I rediscovered myself outside of surrogacy. Only I found that I carried myself differently now; there existed an added dimension to that identity which I called *me*. While I no longer defined myself as a surrogate, my definition of self drew gentle strength from my venture in surrogacy, from giving of myself, from bringing in joy and light and contentment where there had festered devastation and disappointment. I did that. And that became part of me, part of who I could fall back on when I sought self-assurance.

At the end of that first week back at home, Robert and I drove up to

Manhattan Beach for a visit with the new family, leaving the kids in the care of my parents, who had generously remained in town to help out with meals, entertaining and shuttling the kids all around the county to various practices and events. Though promising to stay in touch when they left the hospital, we had not orchestrated a specific agreement with Henry and Lauren on how often we would see each other, preferring to allow that to unfold naturally, mutually respective of our roles in Hope's life and our relationship with each other. Henry and Lauren generously extended us an invitation to visit after settling in those first few days, and I relished the opportunity to witness the impact of Hope's presence in my cousin's home, allowing me another measure of closure on our journey through surrogacy.

And the visit allowed us a chance to hand deliver a cooler full of ex-pressed breast milk with Fed-Ex-like efficiency, friendly door-to-door service to ensure its safe arrival.

"I wish I could suit up and make the delivery in one of those navy blue uniforms," Robert joked mischievously.

When we reached my cousin's house, Lauren and her mom were just returning from a walk with Hope in the carriage for her first visit with the pediatrician, strolling in contentedly with wide smiles on both their faces and Hope fast asleep from the gentle, lulling motion of the stroller sliding over the sidewalk pavement. The doctor had provided Hope a welcome clean bill of health.

"And she wanted me to give you a hug to thank you after she had heard about your role as Hope's surrogate mother," Joyce said, embrac-ing me. Our story it seemed would continue to touch people even after her birth, and that knowledge comforted me; our quest, though over, would not be forgotten.

Robert and I spent a treasured afternoon there in that hushed co-coon that gathers protectively around the arrival of a newborn baby, drawn into the sense of contentment permeating every corner of that space. I noticed a shift in Lauren's manner, a calm and assured claim to her role as mother to this little miracle, within a few short days of Hope's arrival outside of my womb.

Lauren graciously placed Hope in my arms to hold, and as she slept contentedly on my chest for hours, I imparted to her some last words of love and hope and courage for a beautiful life. Though I knew I would see her again, my heart told me that this was the right time to say a final goodbye to my role as her surrogate mother, her protector, so that our connection to each other, though not severed completely by the cutting of the umbilical cord between us, could evolve from the present to a sacred memory of my promise given to her parents to bring her into this world. Though she recognized my voice from her passage inside my womb and her presence in my lap felt so familiar, she no longer felt like a part of me but a part of something we had accomplished together. She belonged now in the loving arms of her parents who had created her and waited for her so anxiously while she took refuge in my belly.

Henry returned home from work early that afternoon, my visit an excuse for him to leave the office and spend time with his new baby girl. Scooping her up immediately when he arrived, he rested on the couch with Hope sleeping on his chest, while we chatted, and I observed him relax into her intoxicating presence, their sense of belonging growing deeper with every rise and fall of Henry's breath.

While he held her I pumped some fresh milk to leave in the freezer along with the contents of the full ice chest we had emptied, several days worth of *liquid gold* in bottles to feed baby Hope. Though I worried that the sight of those bottles of milk which I had pumped from my breasts might cause my cousin some hesitation, he did not appear to exhibit a cooties-like aversion to touching them as he loaded up their freezer before we left; an unusual gift to give and receive, but then he had given me his embryo and I had received that into my body without making any faces. Of course I had not actually been required to touch it. *Nah-nah-na-nah-nah.*

Robert drove me back home to San Diego that afternoon with our emptied cooler; I felt restored and grateful for the opportunity to continue my connection to Hope, comfortable now leaving her and our physical connection behind and following her progress intermittently from a distance. Lulled into a semi-conscious state by the passing freeway traffic, I allowed my thoughts to drift inward, and found myself at peace saying goodbye to the surrogacy after the chance to reaffirm the impact my role as surrogate had played in that corner of Manhattan Beach.

That night back in Encinitas we attended Open House at the kids' elementary school, my first time thrust back into the public arena since Hope's birth. Feeling fragile and unprepared yet to fully engage the outside world, I attended somewhat reluctantly, but recognized my participation as an important first step in resuming the duties of my role as mother of my children, leaving my role as surrogate mother to Hope another step behind. While Kellie and Duncan proudly shared their work and experiences from the year at school with us, my parents were able to witness that night how the surrogacy had touched many people outside the family, as I received dozens of hugs in admiring acknowledgement of the venture I had completed and in congratulations for Hope's entrance into the world. (Some of the congratulations that night came from people surprised to learn only at that moment, when they questioned the whereabouts of the baby, that my pregnancy had succeeded as a surrogacy. The discovery shocked them into silence.)

I had received, in fact, hundreds of extra hugs over the course of the nine months in support of my surrogate pregnancy from friends, family, acquaintances and strangers alike; my body had ached for the emotional and spiritual strength I had received from every single one. The prevailing wisdom suggests you need at least seven hugs a day for maintenance of your well-being, while my own personal research suggested that during surrogacy that number at least doubles. In the end the voyage through surrogacy had emptied my emotional stores, and with almost nothing left inside to give, I could hear the refrain from the Jackson Browne song playing quietly in my head at the school that night, "…….*running on empty*……..".

My body still weakened by the recovery from a surgical birth, my whole being stumbled with exhaustion from the effort of giving up my life for a year to another family. I had dipped deeply into my well of personal strength to manage my worries and concerns about the viability of the baby, to vigilantly monitor the care of my pregnancy, to hold up under the self-inflicted pressure to deliver on my promise to my cousin, and to repeatedly explain my motivations and reassure concerned family and friends of my well-being. Those efforts, combined with the devotion of time a surrogacy quest requires for doctors visits, legal and psychological counsel, logistical preparation etc., and added on to the day-to-day requirements of caring for my own family with three young children, had left me at the end feeling like an exhausted shell of a person, albeit a fulfilled one.

I recognized it would be a process of healing to recover a healthy balance of emotional, spiritual and physical strength to feel ready to give again wholeheartedly and rejoin fully the outside world. With each hug, each word of congratulations, my strength came back to me, not in the flash of a flood, but in a trickle of drops that I would be able to build upon in the weeks to come.

My parents prepared to return home the morning after Open House night, having delivered us a week of respite from the duties of running a household while we recovered from the birth and the surrogacy and made the transition back to our nuclear family. I knew they had been happy to be included in this special moment with their nephew, and they had willingly provided their help and support to make our successful journey a reality.

"Thank you. We couldn't have done it without you," Robert insisted.

"We are so proud of you," my parents both declared, hugging me as they walked out the front door.

A few days later, on Sunday, we piled three excited kids in the car for a trip up to Los Angeles to visit nearly two-week old Hope. They missed their baby cousin and had clamored for another chance to see her, counting her as part of their family now. Cousins often enjoy a special, unique relationship, and in this case the connection between them had developed for months before she even entered into this world.

We all enjoyed a nice quiet day with the cousins holed up in their cozy space as a family, and the kids lit up inside when they were given a chance to hold Hope again and whisper their love to her. Duncan sat still with her in his lap on an overstuffed chair studying her intently for a few minutes, a concentrated effort for a six year old boy, before he pronounced himself *done* and handed her over to jump up and run around outside. For Lise, at three-and-a-half, Hope appeared like a dream of her very own doll come to life, and she smiled like she'd been granted her most special wish when she cuddled Hope in her arms. Kellie, at almost eight years old, admired her cousin lovingly, struggling with a brave face while she held her, wishing, I know, that she could bring her back to our house, yet understanding with a wisdom beyond her years that she did not belong there.

"It is really hard when you love something that normally you would get to keep, but you have to give it up," an insightful Kellie had declared resignedly to me earlier that week, after thinking long and hard about the situation, and comparing it to her memories of welcoming her sister into the family just a few years earlier.

"I know, honey. But it's still o.k. to love her," I had comforted her.

"Mommy, can we take a picture of Hope's room so that I can imagine her there, so that it would make it easier to be away from her?" Kellie asked that afternoon at my cousin's house.

"We can take as many pictures as you want, honey," I answered compassionately, sympathizing with her need to feel connected.

We took a roll of black and white snapshots that afternoon, capturing the affection surrounding a beloved cousin, and those pictures made their way into the rooms of our house and onto the covers of the kids' school binders, one gracing a treasured spot on my desk next to infant photos of each of my own three children. We had traveled to Manhattan Beach that day, it turned out, to say goodbye to that baby growing inside my belly for nine months, and to embrace the new family as part of our extended family, with whom we hoped to visit and share as Hope grows up and takes her place in this world, her cousins cheering her on from the sidelines.

Ten days later on May 31st, my healing from the c-section progressing nicely, I saw Dr. Gerber for my delivery follow-up. Her nurse assistant welcomed me in as soon as I entered the waiting room, and directed me immediately back to the dreaded scale for a post-birth weigh-in. I peeked over her shoulders hopefully as she slid the weights across the scale bars.

Surprise! I weighed six pounds lighter than at the start of the pregnancy. Now I could boast I had returned to my weight before I had carried any babies, and perhaps endorse a new body remodeling program: Become a surrogate and get big boobs, lose your butt, and drop the pesky pounds! (Though there remained that whole belly elasticity tissue issue; the shape of my middle did not exactly resemble the hardened, sculpted six-pack look of my gymnastics days, instead jiggling and expanding in a frightening array of new directions after this fourth pregnancy. Well, no weight loss program is perfect.) What a bonus: I could actually take pride in my post-surrogacy shape.

The nurse, admiring what she observed as my cheerful nature and self-control throughout the surrogacy, questioned me anxiously about my completed surrogacy quest as she led me to an examining room, revealing her own interest in offering to be a surrogate for her sister. I cautioned her that in fact, despite my cheery appearance, there had existed a few times over the last nine months when I temporarily lost control of my emotions and focus, especially during the endless nauseous days of the first trimester and the post-delivery pain. I admitted, though that while I had not begun every day jumping for joy about the practicalities of pregnancy, I rejoiced had daily in its purpose, and overall treasured deeply the journey with my cousin and his wife.

She confessed that she was concerned that the end of a surrogacy might be difficult and emotionally distressing for her, and when she questioned me curiously about my feelings and emotions after the birth, I could sense her concern for giving up a baby. I attested that I had adjusted well, and that, without any regrets, I had felt nothing but thrilled to deliver Hope to her parents, reassuring her that in my case I had never felt in the last year or the last few weeks any remote urge or desire to claim Hope as my own. Simply put, she was not mine, and I counted myself lucky to have claimed my role as her safe haven for nine months so she could make a hopeful couple a family.

"I still wouldn't recommend surrogacy to everyone, because, bottom line, it absolutely is difficult. And you need to be fully committed and comfortable with it," I advised her, though. I suggested that if after researching and contemplating surrogacy she maintained any reservations about the necessary preparation, the long pregnancy, the birth, or delivering the baby back to its parents, she should seriously reconsider whether surrogacy would be the right choice. No sense of desire, duty, or even guilt could be enough on its own to navigate the obstacles and carry off a successful surrogacy.

Dr. Gerber appeared genuinely glad to see me that morning, and when she examined my state of mind as well as my physical health, I assured her that I had reclaimed a portion of my emotional and spiritual strength, and had begun adjusting to life after surrogacy. As she concluded her examination, I thanked her for not only making the practical, medical aspects of the surrogacy so seamless, but also for providing us with her encouragement and emotional support, and accepting our invitation to journey with us through surrogacy as a special privilege.

"Everyone in the office thinks you have done such an incredible thing," she said, looking into my eyes with warmth and admiration.

I smiled in response, not quite sure what to say, not quite comfortable accepting her praise. The truth of it is, though I felt like I had *participated* in a truly incredible thing, and though I had sacrificed to bring Hope to her parents, my role as a surrogate felt like part of a pilgrimage much larger than me. But Dr. Gerber's words did deliver a little boost to my sense of self, to my store of spiritual and emotional strength, adding another drop to the trickle that had begun to heal and restore me.

That night I sat in on another meeting of the surrogacy support group led by psychologist Karen Chernekoff; the same group that I had attended back in October when I had shown up newly pregnant. Seven of us shared our surrogacy stories while we ate a light dinner in a private corner of the same restaurant, and again it appeared that I would be the only one to deliver good news.

Of the ten transfers performed in April on women in the group, an encouraging number of six had resulted in pregnancies (a high percentage), but as of our meeting only two were still viable and one of those appeared to be in danger of failing. And to compound their disappointment was the unfortunate story Karen shared with us about another woman unable to be there that night, who doctors had hospitalized three months into the pregnancy after the twins she carried died in-utero. She and her intended couple were devastated by the loss. (Thankfully that surrogate had known the triumph of delivering surrogate babies successfully twice before, persevering in between a few miscarriages.)

Although none of the women in attendance at the restaurant that night had yet completed a cycle of successful surrogacy, they appeared clearly committed to sticking with it despite the frustration and discouragement of so many obstacles, and I admired them for their desire and fortitude. They so much wanted to succeed for their couples, to be the ones that gave them what they so desperately desired. I had experienced such an easy time of it by comparison! Though, in truth, the last way I would describe the previous year is *easy* after all the time, effort, energy, commitment, pain, and wear-and-tear on my body and mind, still in the end we had succeeded on the first try, and I came to appreciate the blessing of our good fortune even more after sharing my story with other surrogates that night.

I continued to stay in touch with Henry and Lauren by phone every few days as we approached Hope's one month birthday. They were proud, loving parents, and each time we spoke the joy and contentment I heard in their voices reaffirmed our quest of the past year. The emotional distance between Hope and me widened a bit more with each passing day, our connection becoming less present as she bonded deeply with her parents and I thrived on a renewed connection to my own family.

When Henry thoughtfully sent me a videotape of Hope's birth, I relived happily the delivery and our stay in the hospital, all those smiling faces and joyful tears, embracing arms and thankful family, without any sense of loss or any twinge of regret. My heart filled with infinite love and pride, as I watched images of my cousin and his wife overcome with emotion flash across the TV screen.

In the second week of June the final physical insult of the surrogacy descended on my body when I quit pumping breast milk altogether, weaning myself in preparation for our upcoming trip to Kauai. Wrapping my breasts tightly to my body in ace bandages that morning to discourage milk production, I dressed to run a last minute dash to the mall for end-of-the-year teacher gifts.

Midway through the outing my chest ached so fiercely that I could not concentrate, a spreading flame burning through my shirt and piercing my sensitive breasts. Pleading under my breath for the pain to go away, I ditched the shopping and dashed in a café to buy a large cup of ice, racing back to the car with my arms tightly crossed over my throbbing breasts, hoping nobody peered too closely at me. Inside the car I frantically grabbed a plastic bag from the littered back seat, dumping the ice in and holding it directly on my chest, rewrapping the ace bandage haphazardly over the ice bag in a feverish attempt to alleviate the pain driving me to distraction. I had to get home; I was losing it.

Ten minutes down the freeway I moaned in agony and pressed the gas pedal down hard, begging the car to get me home quicker, as the ice leaked through the ace bandage, leaving an embarrassing wet stain on the front of my shirt. I paid little attention to the speed limit, my mind focused deliriously on my goal: a cold shower, a bucket of ice and some extra strength Tylenol waiting for me at home. I almost hoped for an officer to flag me down for speeding, as I fantasized about a police escort home, flying through the fast lane with sirens blaring in front of me. I could not claim the excuse of a life-threatening heart attack, or profuse bleeding, but it damn well felt like a medical emergency to me.

After what seemed an eternity, I finally made it home, stumbling in the door, raiding the freezer and crawling into bed with several ice packs, cradling a bottle of Tylenol; I suffered no long-term damage, but retreated temporarily humiliated by my body's assault, whimpering in defeat.

Nursing myself back to coherency that afternoon while the pain of my engorged breasts receded, I distracted myself with the pretty picture on the dresser in front of me, the arrangement of orchids and anthuriums that stood there brightly, a gift sent from Robert's parents in Hawaii.

The flowers reminded me with their stark elegance of a beautiful passage through surrogacy and beckoned me to embrace our upcoming vacation to Kauai, where I would have an opportunity to complete my recovery and restoration where orchids and anthuriums abound. Though my body had healed almost completely (despite the day's painful relapse) and I had successfully transitioned in large part out of my role as surrogate mom, I looked forward to the time alone with Robert to relax and recharge both physically and emotionally; to enjoy a week suspended outside the obligations of motherhood, a week to reconnect and reflect on our incredible surrogacy adventure and to find some space to try to figure out what might come next.

One full month after Hope's birth, Mom and Dad returned to San Diego, to stay with the kids while Robert and I departed together for a vacation on Kauai, courtesy of Henry and Lauren.

We arrived on the garden island of Kauai in the marbled luxury of the Princeville Resort on the North Shore, orchid leis gently draped around our necks in a Hawaiian welcome. Up in our luxuriously appointed hotel room we looked out on a view framing Hanalei Bay that immediately began to sooth our weary souls. The lush green mountainside rose up across the bay and palm trees swayed in the warm tropical breeze below, where a turquoise pool floated amidst a forest of green umbrellas and chez lounges. The sun caressed our bare skin through the open window, beckoning us to the warm sands for a beachside nap to begin our restoring stay on that garden isle.

That week the healing forces of the ocean waters and the natural beauty that surrounded us, along with the never-to-be-underestimated curative power of a sunset pina colada, served to restore my spirit and to awaken a renewed intimacy with my husband. While we relaxed in the spirit of Kauai, the drops of strength I had gathered since Hope's birth blossomed to a steady stream, like the many pure and clear streams born from frequent rain showers that we crossed on the Kalaulau trail of the North Shore, scrambling up and down the lush undulating cliffs of the Na Pali coastline.

By the end of the week I felt ready to look forward, to enjoy a carefree summer playing with my three children, engaging again in games of tag and baseball in the backyard, splashing in the ocean waves at home, and rolling down the grassy side of a hill when the impulse grabbed me. In that week on Kauai I found my self again, tucked away dormant inside after more than a year focused on a joint surrogacy. And though I largely discovered myself to be the same person I started out at the beginning of that journey, I noticed a subtle twist in my self-perception.

I had given life to a hope, a child, a family, and it had touched me deeply.

When we returned from Kauai, I found Hope's birth announcement peeking out brightly from the pile of banal bills and junk mail I sorted through on the kitchen counter. Smiling in anticipation, I slipped the announcement out of its lined enveloped to reveal a serene picture of baby Hope cuddled into a nest of soft pink blankets. I lovingly traced the outlines of her newborn face with the tip of my index finger, as I gazed at the photograph with tearful pride.

"Hope has arrived into our lives", the card happily announced.

And so, Hope, born of her name, a couple's desperate desire to have a child, had arrived at the beginning of her journey in the world; while I had arrived at the end of our mutual journey through surrogacy, my body and mind intact, with a deep sense of fulfillment and a renewed, expanded appreciation for my children, my husband, my family, my life.

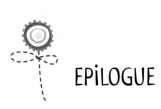

EPILOGUE

Seven months after Hope's entrance into the world, the Holiday season had arrived yet again, but this time without a baby kicking inside my belly.

One morning that December, as had proven true most mornings, I slowly made the rounds to each bed, bleary-eyed and fuzzy-minded, to wake my children from their cozy slumber. Within minutes the sound of opening drawers, running faucets, and feet rushing past to the laundry room heralded the morning's arrival. One by one each of the kids climbed up to the breakfast counter in various states of readiness, crunching on toast, gobbling up melon and swallowing vitamins in haste. Though I am not the cheery, wide-eyed, ready-to-face-the-world type at 7 am, I do my best to make sure the kids are fed, clothed, bathed and nurtured when they stumble into their shoes on their way out the door with Dad before the first bell at school.

The first hour after they leave is my respite, my quiet time alone for reflection, to gear up for the day ahead, and that morning I sat down with my grapefruit, cereal and hot mug of tea to read the newspaper and the mail from the day before. Amidst the pile of Christmas cards from old friends and holiday greetings from various relatives I sorted through that morning, I spied an envelope with a return address from Henry and Lauren. I opened it expectantly.

Inside, I discovered a family photo staring back at me: Henry's family. *Henry's family.* Beaming inwardly, I shook my head in near dis-belief as I cherished the true spirit of the Holiday season before me. The picture illustrated a portrait of love and joy surrounding one perfect pint-size, seven-month-old miracle: Lauren and Henry stood togeth-er on a bluff-top in Hawaii, snuggling in their arms a smiling baby Hope.

I spy a family.

Now that time has passed and my perspective has shifted, I am able to take a closer look at what my journey as a surrogate mother meant to me.

When I carried a baby for my cousin and his wife, I liked to think that surrogacy had some kind of *pay it sideways* effect, where those around me who were touched by the emotional giving that is at the heart of surrogacy would feel inspired to give in their own way to some-one else. After delivering Hope, though, my perspective has changed and evolved. Choosing to become a surrogate mother was a very per-sonal decision and it created a very personal outcome. Can people be touched and inspired by this story? I know that they are. But will it really inspire action? It is probably not likely.

I guess, though, that maybe that is not necessarily the point. Perhaps the more subtle change of focus, the understanding and appre-ciation underlying the conscious discovery of such an act are enough; the knowledge that people can and do choose to take actions that will make a difference for someone else in this disconnected sea of human-ity. Though the story of our surrogacy has perhaps not inspired others to action, it has, in fact, continued to demonstrate the power to touch many people outside our immediate family circle since Hope's birth.

At a baby shower held in Hope's honor, two months after she made her entrance into the world, inside a beautiful home in the suburban hills outside of downtown Los Angeles, Lauren's mother welcomed me in to meet a gaggle of women who had watched Lauren grow up as a young girl, begin a career and fall in love, and who had grieved with Joyce through Lauren's battle with cancer and infertility. There, Lauren and Joyce introduced me to them as the cousin who was *The One*, and each of Joyce's friends thanked me dearly for giving Lauren the opportunity to become a mother, expressing their gratitude with warm hugs and joyful tears, assuring me in hushed, reverent tones that I had changed lives and given a new grandmother reason to hope and laugh again.

I watched proudly as the women passed Hope around that afternoon from one set of embracing arms to the next in the gentle, warm breezes on the coastal hilltop, reveling with inward pleasure at witnessing their awe from the little miracle that had graced the lives of their dear friend and her beloved daughter. I felt honored to claim a role in creating the smiles inspired that afternoon by Hope's appearance, and I celebrated the joy of the event in tribute to the two girls my cousin Henry loved so dearly. And I thought it possible, in that moment, that the appreciation inspired by my generous act could possibly inspire someone else to give generously as well.

The truth is I offered to become a surrogate mother not to change the world, but to help change the lives of my cousin and his wife, to help them create a family. Sympathetic to the devastation caused by infertility, I found surrogacy to be a calling that filled me with excited anticipation, and I can attest to the sense of overwhelming delight accomplishment that I felt in giving the ultimate gift to another couple.

In fact, I would caution any woman considering surrogacy, that the desire to give should be her primary motivation, for there are numerous obstacles to success and it requires a solid set of motivations and expectations to set the foundation for a positive, fulfilling quest.

Making a couple's dream of a child a reality is a worthy goal, justifying and validating all the time and effort required to overcome the legal, medical and psychological obstacles to deliver the happy ending, but it requires personal strength to follow through on the course of surrogacy. I learned that I had to be flexible and willing to make personal sacrifices, and that I had to be prepared to put my life on hold for the benefit of Henry and Lauren and their baby. The unwavering support and understanding of my husband proved to be essential, and I learned that a strong support system is a fundamental necessity for a surrogate to succeed.

Though it is true that any woman considering surrogacy must be prepared to endure the inevitable medical discomfort associated with surrogacy evaluations, tests, hormone shots, the pregnancy itself, the delivery etc., I found that those inconvenient obstacles were manageable because they paled in comparison to the awesome opportunity to follow through on my promise and deliver my cousin and his wife the joy of a family.

Lauren wrote to me in Hope's first year:

I cannot even begin to express the joy that now fills our life. Hope is a true gift from you. We try to cherish every moment with her. I'm amazed at how our lives have changed with her arrival. The love we have for her is overwhelming. It's hard to believe the miracle that brought her here and the amazing gift you have given us.

Lauren is now a mother and my cousin, Henry, is now a father because of our surrogacy. He can walk through the door after a long day at the office to a gigantic little smile that gives him a reason to go back to work again tomorrow. He can scoop up a giggling Hope with his protective hands, hugging and tickling her, knowing that her happiness and *his family* are the only things that truly matter. I know how much that means to them, how much my choice to be their surrogate means to them.

I felt honored and privileged that Henry and Lauren entrusted me with bringing Hope into the world for them, and I appreciated the way they treated me with respect and understanding through their words and actions throughout the surrogacy. I, in turn, included them as much as possible in the joys and realities of the day-to-day pregnancy, and in truth I discovered that the journey centered more on the developing relationship between the three of us than directly with the baby-to-be. So I believe it is crucial that the relationship between surrogates and intended parents is mutually respectful, supportive and trusting, and encourages open, honest communication in order to ensure a rewarding experience.

The privilege of witnessing the birth of a new family in those first hours after Hope arrived, watching Henry and Lauren bond intimately with her, allowed me to appreciate my hard-earned accomplishment as a surrogate mother, and that understanding and acknowledgement ultimately prepared me for the successful transition back to my life after surrogacy. Our frequent communication with each other in the first few days and weeks after the birth provided me with further closure on our surrogacy relationship, their evident joy validated my role as a surrogate and the life-changing adventure we had completed together.

Our families have continued our connection with each other, getting together every couple of months wherever we can over the past several years since Hope was born. At her first birthday party, the power of our quest moved me when the oh-so-normal nature of the celebration (the balloons, the candles, the inevitable frosting all over Hope's face) struck me as truly extraordinary, and that afternoon I held on tightly inside to the pride and joy of knowing that my choice had granted the possibility for that celebration to exist.

Though we do not often discuss the surrogacy with Henry and Lauren anymore, and, in fact, the times when it comes up are fewer and farther between now, still when we are together there is usually a frozen flash of a moment when I am reminded that I helped make her vibrant presence a possibility: a hug or a smile or a giggle that ignites a momentary reverie. Sometimes it's even a comment from Lauren, remarking with a mischievous smile directed toward me, about how Hope's innate love for chocolate must have come from *somewhere else* (all those chocolate chips I ate while she grew inside of me!). Sometimes when they visit us there is someone outside our family around who remembers when I carried her in my belly, and they look at Hope and look back at me and smile with wonder at the outcome of our adventure.

I am so grateful to have had the opportunity to hold out my hand to Henry and Lauren, taking the journey of surrogacy together with them. Surrogacy forged a deeper, more meaningful connection with my cousin that would otherwise have proven unlikely, and I count my friendship with him and his family as a blessing in my life. It is a frequent reminder of what is possible when I choose to participate in life, to hope, to dream, and to initiate the momentum of choices that make a difference, adding permanent meaning and depth to my life's experience.

When Hope grew old enough to understand, Lauren shared the *Miracle of Hope* story with her at bedtime, celebrating her special journey into life. She loved to hear how everyone had joined together to bring her into the world, and every night for months on end she would request the story before finally agreeing to shut her eyes and go to sleep. She has on occasion even proudly shared her birth journey with others in her own words. One morning Hope and her new friend sat buckled into their car seats in the back of Lauren's car on the way to a playdate after preschool, while Lauren spied on them through the rearview mirror.

"*I remember when I was in my mommy's belly, I...*" her friend started.

"*Well, I remember when I was in Pam's belly, I...*" Hope responded matter-of-factly, (much to Lauren's amusement).

Oh, so do I!

While as Hope's temporary surrogate Mom I never felt like her mother, I have always felt a special connection with her. She spent the night with us on one occasion not too long ago, snuggling with Lise into sleeping bags on the floor of her room. When I tucked the girls in, kissed them both good night and turned out the light, Hope spontaneously said for the first time, "*I love you, Pam.*"

I smiled broadly in response, "*I love you too, Hope.*"

I am a treasured cousin now, and though our visceral connection from the pregnancy has dimmed to a subtle glow, our story will connect us together forever.

I entered into surrogacy without huge expectations for the baby I would deliver into the world, because that would have been too overwhelming and unfair to ask of anyone, especially a small child, but I admittedly approached surrogacy with hopes for her, hopes for a bright, happy life, which she is fulfilling every day she wakes up and bounds down the stairs to a wonderful new day. I continue to hope she will find love and peace and adventure, and, in her own way, touch the world around her.

We often celebrate Mother's Day with Henry and Lauren's family, and it is always an opportunity for me to pause to think about Hope and reflect once again on my foray into surrogate motherhood, which is now an immutable, indelible piece of who I am as a mother and an individual. I still have not discovered the secret formula for world peace or the AIDS vaccine, but as I watch my own three beautiful children play with their beloved cousin, I am proud of the joy I brought to Henry and his family through my temporary special role as a surrogate mother.

Our surrogacy is a story of giving, of triumph over adversity, of love, of an affirmation of life.

Each year on May 14th, the day of Hope's birth, a flowering plant arrives on my doorstep from Henry and Lauren in honor of our journey, a reminder that like that plant my gift continues to grow, begun from a seed of life and hope nourished and protected before being delivered. Hope, like that flowering plant, is making her way up in the world, blooming vibrantly, her full beauty appreciated and cherished by those around her.

The flowers always arrive with a card attached that simply says: "Happy Birthday to Me. I love you. Love, Hope".

Happy Birthday, sweetheart.

You can be sure that is one birthday I will never forget.

In Thanks

To the many friends who encouraged me to write this book.

I would like to thank in particular John Moffet and Katie Asch for reading the working drafts. Their guidance and suggestions to dig deeper, write better and share the emotion of my experience helped make it a book worth reading.

Thanks also to Stacey Attanasio for her story perspective and to Deanna Gunn for her insight on publishing a book. Thank you to Kellie, my daughter, who diligently edited each page to fix my many grammatical errors. And to Colette Carlson, Kerry Ojeda, Michelle Gerber, John &Christine Brody, Vanessa Beetham, as well as the Hymettus Ave. Book Club and the Girls Weekend crew, thank you for inspiring me to start and to continue to the end.

I am especially grateful to my husband, Robert, for not only standing strong by my side through the entire surrogacy, but also for reading the early drafts of this book and supporting me in my efforts to finish it.

And, finally, thank you, Henry and Lauren, for not only inviting me to share with you such a beautiful experience in bringing your daughter into this world, but also for your support in pursuing the publication of this book. Thank you, also, to all our families for their love and encouragement.

Me & the
new mom

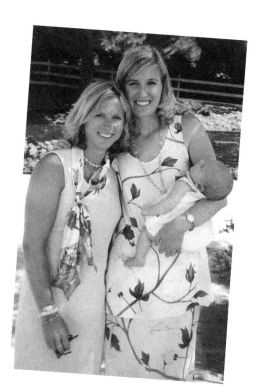

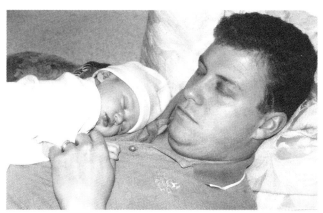

the new daddy

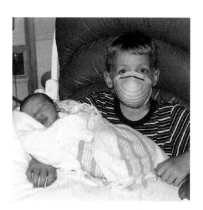

duncan with baby

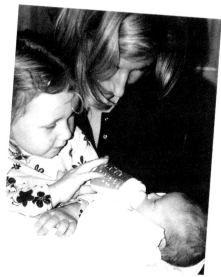

lise & baby
with Lauren

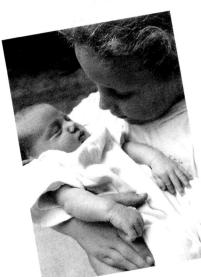

kellie
with
baby

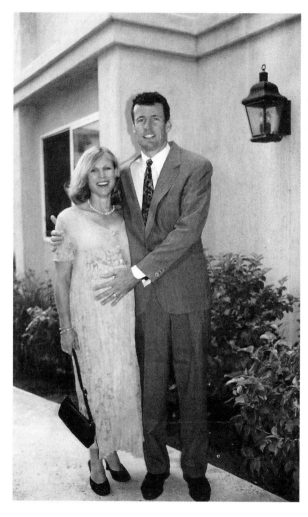

Me &
Robert,
night
of the
wedding

Vist us for more information
and a blog at

deliveringhopebook.com